# THE COMPLETE BOOK
# OF HOME HEALTH CARE

Robert W. Buckingham

*The*
*Complete Book of*

# HOME
# HEALTH
# CARE

CONTINUUM / NEW YORK

RA
645.3
.B83
1984

1984
The Crossroad Publishing Company
370 Lexington Avenue, New York, N.Y. 10017

*Library of Congress Cataloging in Publication Data*
Buckingham, Robert W.
The complete book of home health care.
Bibliography: p. 209
1. Home care services.    2. Self-care, Health.
I. Title.
RA645.3.B83    1984    362.1'4    84-12706
ISBN 0-8264-0350-6
ISBN 0-8264-0352-2 (pbk.)

For my late grandmother
Amelia Rosano Criscuolo
who loved me then
and my children Brandon and Bretta
whom I love now.

# CONTENTS

# PREFACE

Health neither begins nor ends with the physician. The physician's role is important but not as important as that of the consumer. We are all responsible for our own happiness. Health is not a state but a process, and we control the process.

Preventive medicine should be the practice of all. We must try to prevent illness and disease. When disease occurs we must then search out the benefits of modern medicine. But we must remember that not all the components of modern medicine are beneficial. Modern medical institutions are good and bad. They heal but can also hinder health. Not everyone needs institutionalization. Some people heal and recover better at home. Institutions in general are cold, dehumanizing, and degrading to dignity.

It is my belief that home health care is the way of the future. We must realize that home health care can benefit the patient and the family financially. It is significantly less costly to recover from an illness (chronic or acute) at home. Home health care can also benefit the patient and the family psychologically. Patients and their families feel more comfortable at home where they can communicate with each other in more normal ways, and patients always prefer to be at home whenever possible. Finally, home health care benefits the patient physically. Studies show that patients recover quicker at home than in an institution and that there is significantly less chance of infection at home.

We must remember that the American medical system supports dependence upon hospitals and institutions. Hospitals are built for profit and self-perpetuation, for the livelihood and enrichment of management and staff, not for the well-being of patients and their families.

Today there is a paucity of home health care utilization. One out of every five hospital patients today can theoretically get up out of bed, go home, and get better. So I say, go home and get better.

The medicalization of American society must diminish. For far too long the profession of medicine has allowed itself to become overly mystifying, combining aloofness with overpowering authority in a way which produces public disenchantment. It is time we start to take care of ourselves. We cannot afford this foolish dependency on the American medical empire. We must assume the responsibility for our own health and our own illness. We must become informed, educated consumers of the health care system.

As I write this, it is a clear, cool July evening at my summer beach house on Martha's Vineyard. I ponder the fate of this book. Will it be lost on the dusty shelf of some library or will it enlighten people to the benefits of healing at home? I hope the latter.

*Edgartown, Massachusetts*
*July 1984*

# 1

# INTRODUCTION TO
# HOME HEALTH CARE

O ne cold gray wintery New England day, after eighty years of independent living, my great-grandmother fell on an icy road and broke her hip. She was depressed by the prospect of spending months as an invalid in a nursing home while her hip healed, but was greatly encouraged when she learned that with the help of a local home care program she could return to her own home to recover.

At home my great-grandmother healed rather quickly for a woman her age and returned to an active life. Thanks to visiting nurses, a special van that took her to the hospital for checkups, and wonderful meals prepared by friends, relatives, and a part-time homemaker, my great-grandmother was able to resume her lifestyle with her usual good spirits. By April she was able once again to take long walks through neighborhood cemeteries (one of her favorite pastimes).

Home care, as an alternative to costly and prolonged hospitalization or residence in a nursing home, is a growing movement in medicine today. It is being used for patients with such illnesses as heart attacks, which involve a lengthy recovery period; for patients who are chronically ill, for example disabled by a stroke; for patients who are terminally ill; for children for whom a long hospital stay can be extraordinarily stressful; and for the elderly who are too ill or disabled to function entirely on their own.

The American Public Health Association has estimated that at least 10 to 25 percent of the people in institutions could live at home if adequate services were available. Former Secretary of Health, Education and Welfare Joseph Califano has estimated that one in seven patients now cared for in hospitals could be treated as well or better at home.

Ironically, the home care movement is a return to traditional medical practices; until relatively recently, sick and dying people were cared for primarily at home. Prolonged hospitalization was the exception rather than the rule.

## The Advantages

Although prompted more by economics than humanitarian considerations, home care is proving to be emotionally and medically advantageous to patients and their families. Among the benefits that have been noted:

• Wounds heal faster at home since the patient's state of mind, an important factor in recovery, is likely to be much more positive there.
• Patients feel better and eat better when they are surrounded by familiar people and objects and given food prepared to their liking.
• Patients take more responsibility for their own care when removed from the dependency fostered by institutional care.
• Fewer sleeping pills are needed when sleep is not disturbed by unfamiliarity and the noises of hospital personnel and other patients.
• The family is less disrupted by the need to make frequent trips to the hospital.
• Home care costs less.

The kinds of services available at home are expanding rapidly and the number of home care providers, both nonprofit and private, is growing as well. In many communities throughout the country you can participate in home care programs that provide nursing care; transportation to the hospital or physician for periodic treatments or follow-up examinations; rehabilitative therapies, such as occupational, physical, respiratory, speech, and nutritional therapy; counseling by a social worker; medical equipment; various tests and treatments, such as blood tests, intravenous drug therapy, and kidney dialysis; and homemaking services, such as shopping, cooking, and light housework.

Programs vary widely in the quality and extent of services provided and in how much of their cost is covered by medical insurance. Twenty-five states now regulate home health care agencies, and in seven states insurers are required to make home care benefits available to their clients.

Home care is a humanitarian service whose time has come.

## What Is Home Health Care?

Scientists tend to separate humankind's various states into physiological, psychological, sociological categories, and more. These states are further divided into systems and mechanisms of systems. The purpose of this categorization is to simplify analysis and facilitate our understanding of ourselves and the environment in which we live and which we create for ourselves. In health care we find that, although the immediate problem may fall within a particular broad category or may be manifest in a specific system, we must provide a more wholistic philosophy to our care than is implied by the method in which we study ourselves. Home care takes the wholistic approach to client care.

The philosophy of home care places the focus on the patient — his or her needs and well-being. He/she is the center. Any oversight in meeting the posthospital care needs of an individual is considered to be a serious oversight in medication and treatment. Finally, "continuity of nursing" refers to a need for complete cooperation among community organizations, professional personnel, and other citizens.[1]

The very arrangement implied in home care — that the patient receives treatment and comfort at home — is intended to produce a wholistic response from the provider of care. The provider looks at the patient as a whole person existing within the social system of a family and a society.[2] The entire complexity of the human organism and its support structure is considered and employed in treatment.

A more comprehensive definition of home health care would be: ". . . an array of services that may be brought into the home singly or in combination in order to achieve and sustain the optimum state of health, activity, and independence for individuals requiring such services because of acute illness, exacerbations of chronic illness, or long-term permanent limitations due to chronic illness and disability."[3]

Care in the home or a related noninstitutional setting has as objectives three responses to patient care requirements: (1) improve functions to full independence, which ultimately permits the individual to remain at home and care for him or herself; (2) improve or maintain function and enable the individual to remain at home with family or community support; (3) enable a deteriorating person to remain at home as long as possible, when improvement and maintenance are no longer possible.[4]

The purpose of these definitions and objectives is to integrate the idea of home care into contemporary medical care frames of reference. The concept of home care is, of course, not a new one. In societies less advanced than our own, health care has often centered around the family and the home. The desire to integrate these ideas into scientific medical care is not new, either.

The earliest available record of a home care program appears in the fourteenth century in Gheel, Belgium. This still operative program selects families in the community to care for patients as participating members of the family. Originally, the program was created for patients with emotional symptoms.[5]

Early development of home care in the United States came in 1796 with a program for the "sick poor" at the Boston Dispensary. This program still operates on an extended scale.

"Hospital-based coordinated home care programs" began in 1945 at the direction of Dr. E. M. Bluestone of New York's Montefiore Hospital. This was a model of the team concept of care and demonstrated the validity of the inclusion of social workers in the health delivery team.[6]

In Europe, in-home services are widely available and accepted. It is reported that "the proportion of bedfast and functionally impaired individuals living at home is at least as great as the proportion who are institutionalized."[7]

## Home Care versus Institutionalization

As a society, we worship lifesaving activities. Human death is viewed as "a phenomenon to be controlled by machines and active interventions."[8] To a great extent, we don't seem to be geared toward an acceptance of death and the process of dying. Technology-rich hospitals seek to maintain life, or at least life functions, for as long as possible, sometimes without regard to the quality of the life being maintained. There is, on the surface, an implication of passivity involved in the dying process that is intolerable to our medicine and our medical folklore. We fight a nagging feeling that, surely, something can be done to keep individuals alive and that this prospect is much preferable to death. That death itself is manifest and recognized on an intuitive level, rather than simply a rational level, is disturbing to a society proud of its logical understructure.

Family structure has become fragmented, and this nonnuclear social organization has contributed to the trend toward institution-alization. In cases where distance, living facilities, financial limita-tions, or other factors prevent the family from looking after their elderly members, it falls upon the community to provide care. In many cases, however, a lack of services or reimbursement programs for those services makes home care an impractical proposition.

There is no question that a need for home care exists. C. Carl Pegels, in an article appearing in the *Journal of Health Politics, Policy and Law,* reports that 25 to 40 percent of persons institutionalized in the United States today are placed there because of a lack of alternative home health care and community support services.[9] Furthermore, the need for such services in the future is expected to increase dra-matically. In 1975, between 6.8 and 11.8 percent of the population was estimated to be functionally disabled. The total potential de-mand for long-term care services is estimated to have increased from between 5.5 and 9.9 million persons in 1975 to between 6.3 and 11.1 million in 1980 and will reach between 7.4 and 12.5 million in 1985.[10]

Aside from insufficient community care services, the most frequently cited reasons for the overutilization of institutional care include re-strictions under present public programs and the way eligibility for Medicaid benefits is determined. The major barrier to widespread acceptance and utilization of home care services in the United States is the manner in which such services are reimbursed by public and private insurers.

In 1977, the Congressional Budget Office (CBO) estimated the present demand for publicly supported long-term health care ser-vices to be nearly three times the then current supply. Future de-mand was expected to rise 40 percent between 1975 and 1985 (all this for personal care, housing arrangements, home health and day care services). The CBO also estimated that 10 to 20 percent of all skilled nursing facility patients and 20 to 40 percent of all intermediate-care facility residents are receiving unnecessarily high levels of care and "that between 14 and 25 percent of institutionalized patients could be cared for in less restrictive settings (though not necessarily less expensively)."[11] Although the government has acknowledged these high levels of demand and inappropriately high levels of care, it has given Medicare and Medicaid, the driving forces in formation and implementation of long-term care policies for the government, a low priority with respect to reimbursement for home health care costs.

The CBO estimates that over 90 percent of all public expenditures for long-term care go for institutional care. Medicaid is the primary source. In fiscal year 1978, only .8 percent of Medicaid expenditures went for home health care services.[12] Social, homemaker, and personal care support is often excluded from reimbursed home health programs, although these services are seen as crucial by consumers to maintaining life outside a nursing home. A multiplicity of restrictions conspire to make home care an unattractive alternative to the family or individual receiving health cost reimbursement through Medicaid and Medicare.

Private insurance company coverage for long-term care does not generally cover such acute services as extended-care facilities and home health visits. Plans that provide limited coverage for such expenses do so for only limited durations. Home health care is both medical and social. Medical care is "proper" for health insurance programs, whereas social care is not.[13]

If insurance coverage for home health care were made available, the amount of home care sought by persons currently managing on their own is likely to be large. And insurance for home support that defers institutionalization, prolongs life, and increases the quality of life would be highly desirable.[14]

In order to provide the option of home care as an alternative to institutionalization, incentives must be developed for families or relatives to provide care for the elderly. These incentives will be provided by a reimbursement program through public and private insurers that is responsive to the needs of the public. Other incentives promoting home care are well known and could easily provide the sort of market growth required to lure health providers into this field.

The advantages of home care over institutionalization can be very great, depending on the individual requirements of the patient. To be sure, institutionalization usurps from the older person any sense of worth, independence, and dignity. Providers concerned with the chronically ill have maintained for at least a generation that the patient's own home should be used whenever possible as a center for long-term care rather than the often depersonalized institutional set-ting.[15] It is the quality of life that concerns these providers; but the value of this quality, from an economic standpoint, is often debated.

Numerous studies have been undertaken to measure the advantages and disadvantages of home care. To measure the impact of home care services on the utlization of hospital services, a study was made of members enrolled in the Kaiser Foundation Health Plan. The Kaiser Study demonstrated that home care alone did not significantly reduce the cost of acute care for their membership, but that it did contribute to the overall well-being of a significant number of patients. Additionally, home health aides provided 48 percent of all procedures, and the health professionals supervising the program reported that the aides provided effective field service.[16]

A few studies indicate that home care can contribute to the prevention of institutionalization. A multivariate analysis of nursing home utilization found that increases in home health care were associated with decreases in the utilization of nursing homes and "other related facilities."[17]

As health status changes, the economics of home health care (its costs compared to the costs of institutionalization) may also change. A Controller General's Office report to Congress indicated that costs for home health care of greatly or extremely impaired individuals were greater than those of institutionalization. Only about 17 percent of those over sixty-five years of age are greatly impaired, however, and those less impaired could realize savings by being cared for at home.[18]

Once the option of home care is made widely available, the most important question becomes: which persons would receive the greatest benefit from home care and which would better be served in an institutional setting?

Home health care may be indicated if only sporadic care is required. Nonprofessional therapy, meals, and personal assistance, assuming the availability of funding for these services, may be provided quite efficiently in the home. In deciding if an elderly person should be institutionalized, the job of the family, physicians, and social service workers is to make the elderly person aware of the alternatives and probable consequences when transfer to a nursing home is indicated. "If he can comprehend this, whether senile or not, he has the right to decide where he wants to live." If a patient is actively involved in the planning process, he or she will make a responsibile decision regarding care. Authorities caution that evaluations in the hospital may lead to misconceptions of the competency of the patient to decide for or against home care. Disorientation is normally associated with the change of environment and atmosphere between the home and hospital, and the environment of the institution may tend to exaggerate the patient's mental status. The family should seek a wide variety of evaluators and should attempt to involve the ill individual as much as is possible in the decision process. In other words, the same level of concern for the dignity of the patient that precipitated the decision process should be exercised *during* the decision process.[19]

Although much of the current literature is concerned primarily with the long-term care needs of the elderly, home care may admirably serve the needs of chronically ill children and young and middle-aged adults. For instance, a study of a home care program for terminally ill children at the Midwest Children's Cancer Center of the Milwaukee Children's Hospital reported considerable success in the maintenance of function of the ill child and in the bereavement program for the surviving family after the child's death. Pain was controlled as successfully at home as with hospitalized patients, and stress and anxiety were reduced markedly in the home care patients. In interviews a year after the deaths of their child, parents in the program "expressed satisfaction and enthusiasm for their choice of home care."[20] Feelings of guilt and grief over the death were eased, and numerous studies have also concluded that grief is resolved more quickly and effectively when the family is involved with the patient in home care.

## Home Health Care Providers

Home care is provided by hospital-based and hospice-based agencies, visiting nurse associations, public health departments, and private homemaker–home health aide services. Ideally, four social services are provided: (1) case management, where a case manager visits the patient, assesses needs, and provides assistance in obtaining the type and amount of service needed; (2) chore service or home maintenance, in which home cleaning and minor repairs are provided for; (3) homemaker services, such as food shopping and meal preparation; and (4) information and referral services, which help the patient to locate other sources of help.[21] These providers attempt to meet the needs of persons requiring assistance ranging from light, sporadic care to round-the-clock medical care. Such medical care can include physician care and supervision, intermittent skilled nursing care, and physiotherapy.

Hospital-based home health care uses the hospital's care structure over the entire inpatient-noninpatient continuum to insure continuity of care. Medicare programs readily reimburse for services through these programs to patients over sixty-five and Blue Cross and Blue Shield Association coverage extends to intensive and intermediate care categories (those requiring professional coordination of care and active medical and nursing management and those requiring only a single service or a combination of nursing and therapeutic services). It is widely believed that the greatest potential for cost-containment and improved quality of care exists in these two care categories, and studies have indicated an average savings of up to $917 per case through the use of intensive and intermediate hospital-based home care.[22]

Hospice-based home health care programs, particularly those designed for terminally ill cancer patients, concentrate on pain control, acceptance of death as a final phase of life, bereavement counseling for the family, and general quality-of-life improvement for the patient. The unit of care is the whole family, not simply the patient. As provider agencies, visiting nurse associations and public and private services tend to be small and numerous, compared to hospital programs. Quality of service is of foremost concern with these groups, especially private-sector providers. Supervised community living and support services, such as halfway houses, adult foster homes, and protective living arrangements, should be carefully checked before an individual is enrolled in any of them. As financial coverage of home care is expanded, government agencies and consumers should be wary of abuses similar to those that have plagued the nursing home industry.

Social programs must be evaluated in terms of equity, dignity, and cost. The National League for Nursing and the American Public Health Association have instituted a voluntary accreditation program for home care providers. Since 1971 the accreditation program has extended to homemaker–home health aide services, as well as visiting nurse associations. The accreditation process is voluntary on the part of the provider and the final decision to grant accreditation is made by a group of professionals, consumers, and other accredited agency individuals.[23] Such accreditation programs may help to provide the quality controls that will make home care reimbursement more attractive to public and private insurers. Certainly consumers of such services should be aware of accreditation programs.

## Reimbursement and Legislation

As mentioned previously, perhaps the greatest barrier to increased home care services and the spread of acceptance of home care is the manner in which insurance reimbursements for this care are handled. Public reimbursement programs differ greatly from state to state as Title XX permits states to provide a wide range of in-home services and reimbursements through federal Supplemental Security Income. Thirty-four states provide such benefits for state-defined categories of protective living arrangements. In most states, Medicaid home health care benefits constitute .1 to .5 percent of total Medicaid expenditures, but due to the discretionary nature of benefit disbursement from state to state, some states award considerably better benefits to home care recipients serviced in fiscal year 1976 and 81 percent of all federal home health care payments in fiscal year 1977.

In October 1979, the Department of Health and Human Services submitted specific recommendations to Congress, including (1) promoting the development of quality assurance mechanisms for Title XX in-home services; (2) removing the three-day prior-institutionalization requirement for eligibility for in-home care benefits under Part A of Medicare: (3) allowing states without medically needy programs to provide Medicaid coverage for in-home services to certain low-income groups; (4) authorizing the secretary of the Department of Health and Human Services to establish minimum reimbursement levels for home health care under Medicaid; and (5) upgrading skill requirements for all homemaker–home health aides as a condition of participation in Titles XVIII and XIX programs. The effects of this and other actions, such as those that have authorized grants to organizations for the purpose of developing new and expanding old home health care (under the Health Revenue Sharing and Health Services Act of 1975), have only now begun to have an impact on the availability of services and reimbursement for those services.[24]

As the structure of health care delivery in the United States evolves, particularly with the advent of independent physician associations, health maintenance organizations, and such provider-responsible government programs as the Arizona Health Cost-Containment System, consumers may be provided with several attractive home care alternatives.

## Conclusions

Home health care, a long-term care method that takes a wholistic view of the patient's needs and actively involves the family in patient care and comfort, is a desirable and viable option to institutional care (that which is provided by hospitals, nursing homes, and related facilities). Except in some instances of great disability, home care can provide for the patient at costs lower than those of other alternatives to care. Its objectives and operational position with respect to hospitalization and physician care are not abstract — social services can be coordinated with medical services to the benefit of disabled individuals and their families.

Although public and private reimbursement programs have been slow to provide for home care — and the lack of such payment programs have stymied the growth of home care services — this situation is currently being addressed. The need for such insurance coverage is widely acknowledged and will soon be available to a much greater degree than before.

Home care, until fairly recently the only way to provide long-term care, is often ideal for the care of the elderly and for the disabled and terminally ill of all ages. As the health delivery system evolves and education of physicians, social workers, and the public at large continues, the effectiveness and acceptance of this type of care will continue to grow.

It could be said that the important part of "home care" is "care." As a response to a need for better services, the philosophy of home care is based on the notion that the quality of life is determined by the individual and those he or she interacts with closely. Home care is a support group of family, professionals, and the community, which endeavors to provide for the needs of the ill and disabled and contribute to the quality of life for everyone involved in delivering or receiving care.

# 2

# THE HISTORY OF
# HOME HEALTH CARE

H ome health care is an ill person's alternative to hospitalization. Because it offers many advantages, home health care is usually favored by those who have the choice. Some of the advantages are that a patient is able to recover in a comfortable and familiar environment, health care services are provided only when needed, hospital beds are vacant for those actually needing them, a patient's recovery tends to be quicker, and health costs are minimized. According to Earland Cyrus, "Home health care is actually the rebirth of an ancient and honorable concern on the part of the family (in a limited individual sense and also the family in the larger sense of the human society) toward one of its members who is passing through a period of illness. The hoped for end is the restoration to maximum activities of daily living commensurate with the patient's age."[1]

The patient's family contributes to the care of the patient by providing moral support and performing health care duties taught by the nurse. It must be remembered that home health care does not end with the family; friends, relatives, and neighbors can also participate in caring.

The home health care nurse provides medical treatment to the patient and also instructs participants in proper ways of caring for their ill loved one.[2]

The physician plays the role of a manager in a home health care program. It is the physician who changes a proposed program to suit the needs of a patient and then gives the final approval over a program. The physician manages the entire health care plan until the patient recovers. It is also the physician who provides medical care whenever necessary to the patient recovering at home.[3]

There are many other home health care services besides the patient's family, physician, and nurse that facilitate home health care. A homemaker–home health aide performs such duties as cooking, cleaning, and maintaining a patient's personal hygiene. Another service, "Meals-on-Wheels," delivers meals to the patient at home. A patient is usually fed three meals a day—breakfast, lunch, and dinner.[4]

Transportation is another service provided to patients who are unable to go anywhere because of lack of means.[5] Some patients recovering at home need to go to the hospital periodically for medication, tests, etc. Transportation services make this possible.

The Friendly Visitor is a service that provides company to those patients who have no family.[6] The Friendly Visitor is not a substitute, but it does provide the patient with somebody to talk to, watch television with, and, if able, go shopping with.

## The History of Home Health Care

The earliest official home care program known to history was in Gheel, Belgium. Records indicate that this home care program was established in the fourteenth century for those suffering from emotional illness. Amazingly, this Belgian program is still in existence. It operates by selecting families in the community that provide care for the patients.[7] "The providing families," I assume, are on a voluntary basis (service should never be imposed or mandatory). But then again, one must consider that the Belgian people are probably sensitive to the needs of their neighbors and, because of this, have kept this home care program alive through the centuries. I could not see such a program surviving in the United States; Americans are too self-involved.

In the United States, the earliest home care program was established in 1796 at the Boston Dispensary.[8] With the intent of providing medical care to the ill poor, it was based on the following guidelines:

1. The sick, without being pained by a separation from their families, may be attended and relieved in their own homes.
2. The sick can in this way be assisted at less expense to the public than in any hospital.

3. Those who have seen better days may be comforted without being humiliated, and all the poor receive the benefits of a charity, the more refined as it is the more secret.[9]

The first of the above guidelines means that an ill person can be treated at home rather than being institutionalized. One must remember that this depends on the seriousness of the illness and if the necessary equipment is available in the home. The second guideline says that a person can be treated at home at less cost than institutionalization incurs. And the third, that home health care provides an individual the privacy so often lacking in an institution. These early guidelines give one an understanding of the crude basics of home health care.

In the nineteenth century, most ill people were cared for at home. It was usually the mother or oldest female of the household who assumed full responsibility in caring for the ill member of the family.[10] The only time a physician was brought in was when the illness was very serious, so serious that the patient's caretaker may not have known what to do. During this era, the family, friends, and neighbors provided all the help possible—everything from "patient sitting" to moral support. Curiously, all these people play an important role in home health care today.

It must be kept in mind that at this time hospitals were generally thought of as "bad" places to be. They were considered a place for the dying, a last resort. They were also where homeless people and derelicts were treated.[11]

Perhaps those negative feelings were justified. Back in the nineteenth century there were no means of curing such diseases as measles, small pox, and tuberculosis, all of which are so easily prevented or cured today. Proper methods of sterilization were unknown, and a person had a great chance of catching an illness far more serious than the one that precipitated institutionalization. One can only sympathize with the feelings people had about institutions then.

But in the latter part of the nineteenth century, many changes occurred that promoted the development of home health care. For example, in 1875 the Boston University School of Medicine and the Massachusetts Homeopathic Hospital established a home care program that proved so successful it is still used today to instruct medical students in the aspects and techniques of home health care.[12]

Two years after the Boston University School of Medicine and the Massachusetts Homeopathic Hospital added home health care to their curricula the Women's Branch of the New York City Mission was the first organization in the United States to employ a graduate nurse.[13] This nurse was expected to provide nursing care to ill patients in their homes. Thus 1877 marked the introduction of professional nursing care to home health care. The nurses' duties were probably far less than they are today but nonetheless, they were a welcome addition to the growth of home health care.

Other changes that occcured within the next decade (1880–1889) include the introduction of the first nongovernmental (voluntary) home health care agency in 1885. Founded in Buffalo, New York, this agency was to provide organized services to the ill at home. Its main purpose was to provide visiting nurses to the poor recovering at home. Besides caring for the patient, a nurse was also expected to teach cleanliness and proper care of the patient to those involved (family, friends, neighbors).[14]

Because the home health services were voluntary, no financial support existed. Patients were asked to give whatever money they could spare. The success of voluntary home health services was so great that other agencies in Boston and Philadelphia were established in 1886. Soon an association was formed among voluntary agencies providing home health care in the northeastern states, the Visiting Nurse Association. Thus, another asset to the growth of home health care emerged.[15]

In 1898, the Los Angeles County Health Department became the first official health department to hire graduate nurses to provide visiting nursing care to the sick poor.[1] Thus, by the end of the nineteenth century, home health care nursing was begun on the West Coast.

Unfortunately, the latter part of the century also showed a drastic change in the attitudes of people, particularly the wealthy, toward home health care. People felt that having a sick member of their family at home would stifle their social activities.[17] The family probably felt that those invited to their social functions would be in danger of catching whatever disease was being treated, or that the patient required plenty of rest and the noise of the party would only cause disturbance. Whatever the reasons, the wealthy began to discourage care for the sick at home.

During this time, advances were made in medicine that only encouraged the construction of hospitals. Because of home health care disapproval, the wealthy strongly supported and financed hospital construction. But soon after, the poor began demanding better quality of home health care services. This encouraged institutionalization over home health care. Because of this attitude, held by both rich and poor, Americans entered not only the twentieth century, but also a different society than the previous one — an institution-oriented society.[18]

However, the negative attitude toward home health care did not stop its development. Then, as today, people wanted to save money on health care. In 1937 the Hospital Survey for New York recommended that home health care "be developed by the community as an extension of hospital and outpatient service, and that care for the poor be financed by the Department of Hospitals and administered by a full-time salaried physician. Even though home health care already existed under several voluntary hospitals, the use of New York's public funds to finance home health care programs was prohibited by its City Charter of 1901. Several efforts were made, however, and on January 1, 1938, these financial restrictions on home health care were lifted.[19]

Once again the incentive for home health care was so strong that between 1940 and 1942 a study was conducted at the Syracuse University College of Medicine in which a home care program was developed and a group of patients selected to participate after leaving the hospital. The results of the study found that a patient's quality of care was better at home than in an institution, and that this led to quicker recovery.[20]

The next big step in home health care did not come until 1947. This was the year that the first hospital-based coordinated home health care program was established by the Montefiore Hospital, located in the Bronx. The primary objective of its program was to "extend hospital services and facilities beyond the walls of the institution, into the homes of patients who do not require the high concentration of services that is available intramurally." (Intramurally meant within the hospital.) Home care at Montefiore was not to be a substitute for hospital or outpatient care. Rather, its purpose was to treat those patients whose illnesses did not require hospitalization. The Montefiore administrators also realized that by treating patients in their homes, space became available in their hospital for those requiring hospital-ization.[21]

The successful establishment of the first coordinated home health care program led to many other hospital-based programs. For instance, the Montefiore Hospital of Western Pennsylvania, located in Pittsburgh, established its home health care program along the guidelines of the original founder — New York's Montefiore Hospital.[22]

Because this program was successful, the Pittsburgh Montefiore Hospital's board of directors devised and approved a budget in 1961 for a permanent home care department. Although not one of the first hospitals with a home health care program, it still played a major role in the developmental history of home health care:

> With the identification of the home care program as one of five national training centers for home care and related activities, a series of educational programs was developed through seven years of grant support by the Public Health Service. A steady stream of individual physicians, nurses, and social workers, as well as groups of separate and interdisciplinary professionals, came from several states to share this experience. Pittsburgh's Montefiore home care staff engaged in a variety of educational programs, both at their home base through institutes and conferences, and with travel to many other areas to help in initiating coordinated home care.[23]

The introduction of Medicare and Medicaid in 1966 marked a big change in the development of home health care. These two federally subsidized programs were introduced mainly to help those who needed home health care but could not afford it.

Medicare became effective on July 1, 1966. It consisted of two parts. The first, Part A, entitled "Hospital Insurance Benefits for the Aged and Disabled," was devised to provide basic coverage of hospital and related posthospital care costs for the elderly and disabled. It also covers home health care. The cost of short-term, skilled services (physicians, nurses, etc.) for the patient recovering from acute injury or illness are partly covered. To qualify under this part, the patient must have stayed in the hospital for at least three days.[24]

The disadvantage of Medicare is that it only covers short-term home health care under Part A, whereas the main purpose of home health care is to benefit those patients requiring long recuperation periods. And these long recuperation periods are much more of a financial burden than short-term periods. Besides, short-term recovery is usually accomplished in the hospital.

Medicare's Part B helps solve this problem somewhat. This supplement to Part A provides full coverage for costs arising from home health care, such as the physician, nurse, and homemaker–home health aide. It also differs from Part A in that the services must be purchased monthly,[25] so the patient is free to buy any amount desired.

To qualify for Medicare a patient must meet certain criteria. Those eligible for benefits usually fall into one of two categories: over sixty-five years of age and eligible for Social Security benefits, or disabled and under the age of sixty-five who have been disabled for more than twenty-four months. Once eligible, recipients are entitled to coverage for such services as nursing, physical therapy, speech therapy, occupational therapy, medical supplies and appliances, and social service.[26]

The specific requirements of Part A are that a patient must be homebound, hospitalized at least three days, and treatment needed at home is for the same illness as that while institutionalized. The requirements of Part B are the same, with the exception of the mandatory three-day hospitalization period.[27]

Medicaid was enacted under Title XIX of the Social Security Act at about the same time as Medicare. Under this program there are funds that are specifically allocated for home health care. Under Medicaid, the federal government requires that each state devise and administer its own home health care program plan. Plans differ from state to state. The services an eligible patient receives are the same as with Medicare, the only difference being that eligibility cannot be based on whether a patient was institutionalized before home health care was recommended. This is advantageous because it minimizes home health care costs from the start by not requiring costly institutionalization in order to qualify. The disadvantage is that in many states reimbursement to the patient is very low, costs of care far exceed the reimbursement amount, presenting potential financial burdens on the home health care patient.[28]

Medicare and Medicaid have not had the results expected in helping patients with financial problems:

Medicare statistics show that in 1969, 1.3% of the $6.25 billion Medicare budget (or $85 million) was spent for home health care. Six years later, while 25 million persons did receive home health services at a cost to Medicare of $250 million, that figure still comprised a mere 1.5% of the total Medicare budget of $16 billion. Medicaid statistics are equally discouraging. In 1967, only 0.9% of the total Medicaid budget ($28.9 million dollars) was spent in home health care; in 1973 this was reduced to 0.7% of the total budget, or $63.8 million.[29]

Instead of contributing to the development of home health care in this country, these programs actually slowed its growth by allocating such a small amount of funds.

Today there is much happening in the field of home health care. For instance, the federal National Health Planning Act is being developed to increase the quality of health care and, at the same time, to minimize costs as much as possible. How this affects home health care can be seen from the following statement: "Increases in the cost of health care, particularly of hospital stays, have been uncontrollable and inflationary, and there are presently inadequate incentives for the use of appropriate alternative levels of health care, and for the substitution of ambulatory and intermediate care for inpatient hospital care."[30]

Home health care is a good alternative to the high costs institutionalization imposes on a patient. Unfortunately, "inadequate incentives" discourage home health care. More money from Medicare and Medicaid should be used to subsidize home health care. Not only will this help those patients unable to afford and obtain it, but it will encourage many potential home health care participants to consider using it. Everybody wants to save money, and home health care is a significant way to do so.

Considering the benefits that do exist for home health care, its growth in the past ten years has been slow. As mentioned before, lack of government and private programs for funding is one significant reason. Most people refuse to pay the full costs of health care and others simply cannot afford to. Another factor is that home health care services tend to be located in wealthy areas where money is available to support it, but not in low-income areas where people really need financial support.[31]

Another reason for slow growth has been the type of programs shown on television. Shows involving hospitals are usually centered around the institution.[32] This causes most viewers — a great proportion of the American public — to think that everything involved with health care takes place within the hospital. The media should show a little more responsibility in educating the public to this vital aspect of health care.

Physicians are also to blame. Because of the lack of information concerning home health care, many physicians find it uninteresting. Others feel that home health care would only increase their workload. Still other physicians feel that home health care would change the traditional patient-doctor relationship.

## Conclusion

Home health care is made up of many elements. The main care providers in a program are the patient's family, nurse, and physician. The family plays a very active role in home health care as compared to in institutionalization. The family contributes by maintaining the morale of its ill loved one. This is possible because the family knows what the patient's personal needs are and is able to meet them. The family also participates by actually treating the patient, using methods learned from the nurse, such as how to handle a bedridden patient to maximize comfort and cleanliness.

The nurse provides health care. Duties include giving necessary medication at appropriate times and monitoring a patient's recovery progress. It is the nurse who advises the physician of any changes so that the health care program can be modified. The nurse, as mentioned above, also provides instruction to the family in methods of caring.

The physician provides medical care to the ill patient whenever necessary. In home health care the physician also manages the patient's program until recovery. The physician modifies and approves a home health care program, based on the information supplied by the nurse.

Throughout the centuries, home health care has had to struggle just to exist, and even today, it is still in its infancy. If home health care is going to grow, it must be widely accepted by all involved. Physicians must be better informed of its benefits and must consider it an asset to the health profession. The media must share the responsibility by providing information on home health care to the public; this includes television programs and newspaper and magazine articles. The federal programs Medicare and Medicaid must allocate more funds for home health care, instead of the inadequate amount now allocated. But the main responsibility lies with the people themselves—people who are looking for ways of minimizing health care costs, people who are looking to better their quality of health care. *The main responsibility for our own health rests with us all.*

Health care has come full circle in its history by returning to home health care. It is only logical when one considers the cost in money, time, and resources to keep someone in the hospital. The improvements in medical knowledge and technology have overshadowed home care. But despite improving medical and nursing facilities, the home is the primary place for care. Hospitals are gearing more toward acute patient care to cut costs and decrease the need for expansion. With governmental financial support, home care is more accessible to the public.

Yet the most important factor in home care can be found in its name. The *home* fills the physical and spiritual needs of the sick, because it offers a sense of security and normalcy when it is most needed. The home is the traditional place of health care. Given the limits of medical resources, home care is a tradition that works.

# 3

## LEGISLATION AND HOME CARE SERVICES 1935–1982

H ome care in the United States is growing in scope and demand. The increase in home health agencies stems from years of legislation that increased incentives for home care expansion in the health care system. This chapter will examine in depth the fundamental legislation and the history of home care legislation beginning in 1935 with the passage of the Social Security Act and ending with the Tax Equity and Fiscal Responsibility Act passed in 1982. Not until the last two decades has new legislation directly affected the increase in the home care sector services and agencies.

### Early Legislation—The Social Security Act of 1935

During the Great Depression, when Franklin D. Roosevelt was president, there was a strong need for social reform. America had to develop an extensive system of public assistance and a form of social insurance. There were many debates over whether or not Congress should establish a national insurance program. In 1935, the Social Security Act was passed, setting a precedent for further legislation. Initially, there were no provisions for home care. The act established three categories of public assistance program: for the aged, for the blind, and for dependent children. Under this act, the states and the federal government were to establish and administer the program finances. Services were to be covered by federal government matching funds with the individual states that were participating in the program. Although there were no provisions for home care, this legislation was monumental because it established the country's first social insurance program. "It represented the first major entrance of the federal government into the area of social insurance and it greatly and significantly expanded federal grant-in-aid assistance to the states."[1] This act formed the basis for future health programs such as Medicare and Medicaid.

## Legislative Amendments of 1939 to 1963

From 1939 to 1963, there were many debates over what types of services should be offered or covered by the Social Security Act. Several amendments were enacted that enlarged the scope of the provisions. In 1939, the Social Security Act was broadened to include benefits for survivors and dependents.

## Legislative Amendment of 1950

In 1950, federal assistance was extended further to include permanently disabled persons under Title XIV. The federal government matched payments for medical services to the states for all persons in need. Now the public assistance categories included:

• Old Age Assistance (OAA)
• Aid to Families with Dependent Children (AFDC)
• Aid to Blind (AB)
• Aid to Permanently and Totally Disabled (APTD)

## Social Security Amendments of 1960

This was also known as the Kerr-Mills Act. The most important provisions of this amendment were for medical services for the aged. The act was passed after extensive congresssional debate concerning establishing health insurance for the aged. Title I of the Social Security Act was amended to read "Grants to States for Old Age Assistance and Medical Assistance for the Aged." The name change took into account the new policy of having the states provide medical assistance on behalf of aged individuals who were not recipients of Old Age Insurance, but whose resources and income were not sufficient to meet the costs of necessary medical services. "This established a new program of Medical Assistance for the Aged (MAA) providing for federal aid to the states for payments for medical care for 'medically indigent' persons age sixty-five and over." Now a broad range of medical services could be made available. This amendment stipulated the inclusion of institutional and noninstitutional care. The Kerr-Mills Act was the forerunner of Medicaid. Potential services to be covered were inpatient and outpatient hospitals or clinics, nursing homes, and very limited home care.[2]

## Social Security Amendment of 1965/1966—The Advent of Medicare and Medicaid

Until 1965, the most prevalent problem with the Social Security System was that states could determine the extent of services and the conditions of eligibility for such services. "The overall national problem of adequate medical care for the aged has not been met to the extent desired under existing legislation because of the failure of some states to provide coverage and services to the extent anticipated."[3] A new program was needed. The 1965 Social Security Amendment was the answer. It established Medicare, the culmination of many years of congressional debate. It was of great historical importance because it defined and set guidelines on home care services. The amendment also included expanded provisions of the Kerr-Mills Medical Assistance Program to the elderly, known as Medicaid.

Health Insurance for the Aged (Medicare) was added to the Social Security Act (SSA) under Title XVIII. It was divided into two main benefit packages: Hospital Insurance Part A and Supplemental Medical Insurance Part B. Both benefit packages will be discussed in depth.

### Part A: Hospital Insurance Benefits

Under Title XVIII, this insurance program provided basic protection against the cost of hospitals and related posthospital services:

• Posthospital extended care, such as nursing homes, included one hundred days of paid service during a spell of illness. It is important to note that to receive federal funds, a person first had to be put in the hospital before receiving nursing home or home care benefits.

• Posthospital home health services were included and rather limited. This act only provided payment for services for up to one hundred visits in a one-year period.[4]

The amount payable for these two types of services, except home health care, were subject to a deductible and coinsurance payments by the beneficiary. The conditions for payment had provisions to provide service for posthospital home health services. Certification was needed and required if the individual was confined to his or her home and in need of skilled nursing care, physical or speech therapy for conditions for which he or she was receiving inpatient hospital services. "Services must be rendered under a plan made by the patient's physician within fourteen days after his/her discharge from the hospital or extended care facility."[5]

### Part B: Supplementary Medical Insurance

This is a voluntary insurance program financed by premium payments from enrollees and contributions from federal funds. Benefits consist of home health services up to one hundred visits in a one-year period. The conditions for payment include certification by a physician that the individual is confined to his or her home and needs skilled nursing care, physical or speech therapy, and that the services are furnished while the individual is under the care of a physician.

### Part C: Definition of Home Health Agencies and Services

A home health agency is defined as an organization that:

• primarily engages in providing skilled nursing services and other therapeutic services
• has policies established by a group of professional personnel, including one or more physicians and one or more registered nurses, and provides for supervision of such services by a physician or a registered professional nurse
• maintains clinical records on all patients
• if in any state providing for the licensing of this nature is so licensed or meets the licensure standards[6]

Home health services were defined as the following items and services furnished to an individual under the care of a physician by a home health agency on a visiting basis in an individual's home:

• nursing care provided by or under the supervision of a registered professional nurse

• physical, occupational, or speech therapy
• medical social services
• home health aid services
• medical supplies and use of medical appliances
• any of the foregoing provided on an outpatient basis at a hospital, extended-care facility (ECF), or rehabilitation center that involves the use of equipment that cannot be made readily available in the home[7]

Posthospital home health services could be furnished to an individual within one year after his or her most recent discharge from a hospital in which he or she was an inpatient for not less than three consecutive days, or from an extended-care facility. In either case, the plan for home health services is to be established within fourteen days after such a discharge.[8]

Home health visits must be supplied by or through a home health agency. This may be a public agency or a private, nonprofit organization primarily engaged in providing skilled nursing and other therapeutic services. The agency must be governed by policies established by a particular professional group, which includes at least one physician and one registered nurse.[9]

Even with all the changes in legislation, the incentives in the health care system led primarily to institutionalization, as demonstrated by the hospital requirement prior to establishing home health services. Gradually, with the establishment of new legislation, this incentive has disappeared. It is important to note that Medicare has not only enabled the elderly to get more health care, but it has undoubtedly improved the quality of care received. "Qualitative improvements have been most apparent in the area of extended care and home health services, both of which barely existed before Medicare."[10]

## Social Security Amendment of 1967

This amendment extended payment for physical therapy furnished and supervised by a hospital or by other approved providers, whether performed in the patient's home or in an outpatient clinic. The legislative movement is toward providing more home care for those who actively seek the home care option as opposed to being institutionalized in a hospital or, worse yet, a nursing home. It was recognized that "in certain instances, patients of a hospital or ECF may have progressed to the stage where they could be cared for at home with a certain minimal amount of services, which are generally referred to as visiting nurse services or home health services." The home health services included not only visiting nurse service, but also part-time service of a home health aide (not solely for housekeeping purposes), medical supplies and appliances, and the services of interns and residents in training at hospitals within the home health agency. Under the inpatient hospital and ECF benefits, there was a requirement established that stated that an individual must have been hospitalized for a least three qualifying days, and that the home health service plan be established within fourteen days after discharge. In this example of reimbursement for services institutionalization limited the home health services to those individuals who were hospitalized.[11]

Since Medicare and Medicaid were the primary reimbursement programs, they severely limited the home care system in the 1960s. "Funding for home care is very fragmented," says Ann Carter, director of Ebenezer Community Services, "because of limits on the kinds of services available under Medicare. Most agencies that provide anything beyond services reimbursed by Medicare, as the Ebenezer Society does, usually have a funding package that includes private foundations, contributions, home agency subsidies, and client fees."[12] Medicare is behind the times in its policy on reimbursement of home care agencies. Medicare regulation now only reimburses home health aids who perform limited personal care and domestic duties.

Under Social Security Amendment Title XVIII (Medicare and Medicaid), it was important to be certified as a home health agency in order to receive Medicare reimbursement. "The number of community-based units and agencies providing home health care services expanded, but hospital-based programs remained stable in number. From 1966 to 1977, the number of Medicare-certified home health agencies doubled. But the home care emphasis changed, and the coordinated multi-disciplinary long-term care approach was muted. Home health care was seen as short-term, 'skilled' service primarily for the elderly, with many limits placed on visits and services. The chronically ill and disabled younger adult did not fit in."[13]

When Medicare was enacted, it seemed likely that there would be a considerable shortage of home health agencies and certainly a great disparity among different areas, especially outside large cities. An intensive drive was made to stimulate the establishment of new agencies and to strengthen existing agencies so that they could qualify to participate. At the time of inception, about twelve hundred agencies qualified to participate in the Medicare program, and in the next two years this total increased to about twenty-one hundred. About two-thirds were divisions of local health departments.[14] The home health system was stimulated to grow, but still needed to be reformed in order to expand services to meet the demands of the elderly, disabled, and chronically ill. Steps are being taken now to examine and expand Medicare reimbursement and thus increase home health services. There are many reasons for the increased demand in home care agencies: the growing elderly population, improved third-party reimbursement policy, more chronically ill patients who want to be at home, and an increase in public awareness of home care.

## Social Services Amendment of 1974

Title XX, Grants to the States for Services, was added to the Social Security Act in 1974. The act stated the goals of the program, which included the "prevention of inappropriate institutional care through community-based programs."[15] A wide spectrum of social services could be provided, including homemaker services and home-delivered meals.

Then in December 1977, President Carter signed into law a bill that authorized for the first time Medicare and Medicaid payments on a cost basis for services of physicians' assistants, nurse practitioners, and nurse midwives, thus extending home health care services even further.[16]

Legislators have to make changes to reverse the incentives that now reward nursing homes according to the extent of a patient's disability. Nonphysician practitioners have also been able to raise to a new level an area of care that has largely been abandoned by physicians — home care services.[17]

## The 1978 Definition of Home Health Services

The term "home health services" describes an array of services — both therapeutic and preventive — that patients in their homes or foster homes receive for acute illness or disability. A coordinated home care program, centrally administered and through coordinate planning, evaluation, and follow-up procedures, provides physician-directed medical, nursing, social, and related services to selected patients at home.[18]

One study matched two groups of patients—one in a hospital and the other in a home care setting—and found that the results of care did not differ significantly. It indicated that home care is an acceptable alternative to hospitalization. "Organized home care can reduce patient costs, the effect of institutionalization (particularly 'transplantation shock' for the elderly), and the effects of isolated or neglected care. Hospital home care programs can free hospital beds and reduce the average length of stay." Those over sixty-five are the fastest growing "minority group" in the United States, and by 1990 they will increase by another 25 percent. They are also the largest single group of chronically ill. Therefore, legislators are beginning to recognize the demands and needs of the elderly.[19]

## The Omnibus Reconciliation Act of 1980

The Omnibus Reconciliation Act was enacted in 1980 to stimulate future growth of home care agencies by reimbursing for more benefits. This act reflected the concern of legislators to contain costs and enhance efficiency in the Social Security System. "The home health services provisions were revised to remove the one hundred visit per year limit for both Parts A and B, to eliminate the required three-day hospital stay for visits under Part A and the deductibles under Part B."

The need for occupational therapy was made a possible qualifying criterion for initial eligibility for such home visits. This act states that proprietary home health agencies could participate in Medicaid in states that licensed home health agencies since occupational therapy was eliminated. State Medicaid programs were required to provide payment for services by nurse-midwives, if they are legally authorized to perform in the state.[20]

This legislation incorporated extensive budget reductions and program revisions. Particularly notable were the consolidation of a number of programs into three block grants to the states. These were for preventive health services, home health agencies, and public health services.[21] Now there is no limit on the number of annual reimbursement home visits, no longer a $60 home care deductible, and no state licensure requirement for profit agencies that want to participate in the Medicare program. These changes have established home care as a necessary part of the health care delivery system.

## Tax Equity and Fiscal Responsibility Act of 1982

The Tax Equity and Fiscal Responsibility Act has had a big effect on health care providers. There are three main sections of this bill that are instrumental in creating changes in the health care system.

Section 101 has tightened the limits of inpatient service provisions of Medicare to hospitals. This established a limit on the amount of money Medicare will reimburse the hospitals, and it puts the hospitals under pressure to hold costs within those limits, perhaps by decreasing the length of inpatient stays. Hospitals will have an incentive to try to decrease costs as they come close to the ceiling amount. There is another incentive that "takes the form of a 'bonus' to hospitals whose operating costs are below the annual target rate established for Medicare payments." Hospitals that are under the prescribed target rate will be reimbursed for what costs were incurred and 50 percent of the difference between the costs and the target rate established. The opposite is also true; Medicare will penalize hospitals that go over the target rate plus 25 percent of costs in excess of the target rate. Also in Section 101 is a provision for a prospective payment system for skilled nursing homes, hospitals, and other providers. "The theory for using a prospective system is that if health care institutions and other providers are reimbursed at a predetermined rate and allowed to retain any savings for less, the delivery system should become more efficient and cost-effective."[22]

Section 102 deals with single reimbursement for health care agencies. Because of the reasoning that hospital-sponsored home care agencies incur higher costs than independent agencies, it is a blow to hospital-sponsored agencies. A single-payment limit is established based on the experiences of independent home care agencies. The bottom line states that hospital-sponsored agencies' Medicare reimbursement has been decreased. "Hospitals should consider re-organizing their home care program as an independent agency located in or near the hospital."[23] It is important not to eliminate the advantages of having a home care agency staff as part of a hospital team as well.

Section 122 extends Medicare benefits to services that are already available to individuals; that is, hospice care for the chronically ill. Under Part A of Medicare, hospice care for the terminally ill is covered if the patient has under six months life expectancy. Benefits have included traditional nursing care, medical social services, short-term inpatient care, medical supplies, and counseling services for the patient and family. If a hospital wants to establish a hospice extension of services, it must seek additional certification as a hospice provider to receive any Medicare reimbursement.

Section 131 establishes copayment by Medicare recipients. Many states now require some compensation from the individual to cover a part of the expenses that are incurred. Health care providers have to offer a service regardless of the patient's ability to pay or not, thus establishing a larger debit. "Reimbursement units to home health agencies allowable for services are now reduced from 80 percent to 75 percent."[24] Medicaid regulations have contributed to high rates of institutionalization by discouraging the use of community services, although this is changing. The new law allows states to include non-medical community services as a coverable item.

Overall, this law is a "welcome change," says Dr. Robert Kane, director of Geriatric Medicine at the University of California. It is questionable, however, whether states will want to invest the time and money needed to support community-based services. "If a state chooses to apply for a waiver to provide home and community, the standards for assessing the recipient's needs for care, as well as the development of eligibility criteria, will be major factors in determining the benefits of such a program."[25]

The new changes in Medicare and Medicaid will provide the financial supports for those who cannot afford medical care and at the same time will create incentives for hospitals to cut costs. "Medicare might save millions of dollars by reimbursing for respite care at a fraction of the cost of maintaining an elder in an nursing home." Now is the time for new legislation to meet the demands of those in need, whose only alternative to institutionalization is the establishment of home care agencies throughout the United States. In the past the Medicare system favord institutionalization. Medicaid in 1977 covered total costs of indigent nursing home care; it paid $7 billion in such costs, but only $179 million for home health programs. "An astounding 25 percent of the Americans in nursing homes do not have to be there," says Representative Claude Pepper, who heads the House Select Committee on Aging. "They could receive less costly care at home." Home care is in demand and has to be addressed by the state and federal legislators to ensure that the quality of life and the home care option for individuals is met.[26]

The future trends in home care agencies look very positive in the form of expansion of services. With new findings, such as a decrease in mortality for those individuals who are at home and the impact of patient and family counseling, the need for home care is apparent. Society's attitudes are changing toward home care. People now seem to appreciate an option that allows the family to be with the sick family member and to share the last months together in a comfortable, familiar setting.

In the future, hospitals will be forced by Medicare's financial incentives to establish their own home care agency, maximizing profits for the hospitals and providing needed care by extending their resources. "Home health care now is being recognized as a vital service for acute care patients, and increasing numbers of hospitals are developing home health care programs as a direct service to their patients."[27] Hospitals have to become more involved in the home care system, but not lose sight of the primary purpose of providing this type of service for it to be effective.

Many changes have occurred in home care legislation since 1935. During the Depression many Americans could not afford medical services, thus the demand of a social insurance program. Although there were no major provisions relating to home care services directly, the act set in motion the expansion of services and included home care as a necessary part of the health care system.

Similarly, in the 1960s the Kerr-Mills Act extended medical provisions for the aged and set the precedent for Medicare and Medicaid. Up until then, there was a strong incentive to institutionalize, rather than to utilize home care services. Most elderly people found themselves in nursing homes and hospitals before they died.

It was not until 1965, with the advent of Medicare and Medicaid, that Social Security Insurance rapidly started to provide more services to more "needy" individuals, with a concomitant increase in expenditures for the states and the federal government. Part A, the hospital insurance benefits, included posthospital extended care, such as nursing home facilities, for up to one hundred days of paid service.

Again, institutionalization was stressed in practice; an individual had to have been hospitalized before home care benefits would be authorized. The coverage extended to one hundred visits in a one-year period. Part B, the supplemental medical insurance, required those who enrolled to share some of the expenditure costs. The coverage it gave amounted to one hundred visits of home health care, contingent on the individual's physician recommendation. This insurance included provisions for physical and speech therapy at home.

In 1967, legislators found more evidence that home care was just as effective and much more effective than hospitalization or nursing home facilities. The states set the standards and criteria for what could be certified as a home health agency. An agency had to meet these criteria to receive any reimbursement under the Medicare and Medicaid program.

In 1978, home health services expanded its definition to include therapeutic and preventive services at home. The Omnibus Reconciliation Act of 1980 stimulated further growth by reimbursing for still more benefits, thus creating an incentive for home health agencies to expand their services. For example, an occupational therapist was eligible under Medicare. The licensure process for home health agencies were eliminated and midwives were not eligible for coverage provided under the Social Security System.

The Tax Equity and Fiscal Responsibility Act of 1982 tightened the limits on medical hospital provisions because of the skyrocketing costs associated with hospitals. Today there is a strong need to be concerned with cost-containment rather than access and quality. The home care system incentives are changing, due to the new reimbursement program for hospitals. Hospitals now have to watch costs or they will be penalized. The same type of cost control was instituted for hospital-sponsored home health agencies, since they too have a record of exorbitant costs. This act also provides for home services to be covered for the "medically indigent." Future legislation will continue to regard home health care as a viable option in the health delivery system.

# 4

# THE PSYCHOLOGICAL EFFECTS
# OF HOME CARE

T oday more and more people are realizing that institutionalization is not the only way to take care of our sick, disabled, and elderly populations. In fact, it may not even be a very good
way to care for these people as total human beings. People are now
looking for alternatives to these sterile, impersonal institutions, and
they are finding that home care is a good answer. Home care of the
patient, either by a special nurse, friend, or family caregiver, provides
many psychological benefits to the patient, and this is especially true
of the very old, the very young, and the dying. At home, the patient
can be treated as a "total" person and not as just an illness. More time
can be spent with the individual to get to know his or her real needs.
The patient is in familiar surroundings and is therefore more comfortable and less stressed.

Home care also has a great number of psychological effects on the
patient's family. Taking care of a sick, disabled, or elderly person can
be very difficult and stressful for the family, but it can also be a psychologically rewarding experience. With the support of home health
care teams and close family and friends, home care can be a beneficial
experience for everyone involved.

There are psychological costs and benefits of home care, but the
benefits seem to prevail and make home care a desirable alternative
to institutional care.

## Home Care—Psychological Benefits for the Patient

Until recently, institutionalization in either a hospital or nursing
home has been the only choice for someone who is incapacitated by

illness or for the elderly who can no longer care for themselves. Many of these institutions provide good physical and medical care, but their emotional and interpersonal sterility can destroy all zest for living and even the will to live.[1] Many people now realize that the psychological benefits of an alternative to institutional care — home care — can greatly facilitate the physical and mental well-being of these people and especially those who have a devoted and loving family to care for them.

Whatever the condition and the prognosis, the length and the quality of life remaining to the sick or injured person depends greatly on the interaction of his or her personality and overall medical, environmental, and emotional support. In an institution, the patient loses a tremendous amount of independence and self-identity. There is an elaborate division of labor and no one person is really acquainted with the patient. No one has time to talk to the patient and find out what the patient really needs. New technicians and nurses are constantly coming in and administering new procedures with new apparatus, without explaining what's going on. Patients are often treated more like an object than a person. Things are done to the person's body to help it medically or to make it physically more comfortable, but often without even speaking to the patient. These and many other aspects of institutionalization cause the patient a great amount of anxiety, stress, loss of responsiveness, and depression. This is hardly a beneficial environment in which to facilitate the patient's physical or mental recovery from illness or accident.[2]

Contrast this to home care, where the person can be at home surrounded by his or her personal belongings and, if possible, loving family members. At home, the person can be treated like a respected and loved person, not just another case. One-to-one patient care either by a nurse or family member allows the caregiver to know the patient well and adapt to the patient's emotional as well as physical needs. Instead of doing things to the patient or for the patient's body as an object, the caregiver can take time to do things with the patient, with the patient's enjoyment, understanding, cooperation, and help. This one-to-one care at home can reduce stress and be stimulating, instead of depressing, as the multiple impersonal contacts in the institution often are. Also, the continuity of home care makes it possible for the patient to know what to expect, to get accustomed to the nursing procedures, and to be free of the anxiety that is often aroused in the institutional setting, where there are so many unfamiliar workers coming and going.[3]

At home the patient also has the independence to decide when to get up in the morning, when to shave, when to have a bath or a shampoo. He or she can decide when to have visitors and how certain medical routines are carried out. Many choices can be made by the patient at home, and even minor choices enhance one's sense of autonomy. It is crucial to nourish the patient's sense of competence and encourage the making of choices about every possible aspect of one's life. This can only be done in a home setting.[4]

Patients want to feel like persons and have a great need to reestablish their familiar self. When one is stricken by an illness or a major accident, there is an immediate and pervasive feeling of having lost an important part of oneself and being cut off from all closeness with another person through any type of sexuality. As long as one is institutionalized this is true; but at home the possibility of expressing intimate feelings does not need to vanish with the illness or disability. Even when intercourse is no longer possible, affectionate touching, hugging, and kissing can enhance the patient mentally and physically. There is a lot of healing in the magic of love.

At home, those who love and understand the patient have the best chance of restoring emotional balance, of evoking trust and hope, and of stimulating the patient to mobilize all of his or her physical and psychological resources, both to cope with stress and to cooperate in rehabilitation.[5]

An example of the psychological benefits of home care can be seen in the case of the hemophiliac child. A chronic disease such as hemophilia is often a major deterrent to normal psychological development. Studies have shown that there appears to be a direct relationship between the lack of psychological development and the sense of helplessness experienced by patient and family in the face of illness. The more powerless they feel to deal with episodes of bleeding, the more likely the hemophiliac will respond with dangerous behavior or unnecessary passivity.

Home therapy seems uniquely suitable to promote realistic self-care, and it may facilitate development by lessening the sense of helpless dependency upon the hospital. Patients are enthusiastic about home care and report improved performance at school, greater freedom, and more social activity. Home care decreases the time the patient spends in the sick role and allows more time for age-appropriate activities. There is less fear of the consequences of normal physical behavior and less parental concern about fragility and vulnerability. These reponses will be a positive influence toward normal psychological maturation. Home care offers considerable promise in promoting greater independence and freedom for the patient, thus promoting psychological development and well-being.[6]

## Psychological Effects of Home Care on the Aged

Each year thousands of elderly people are moved from their own private environment to an institution; for most, this move is final, since the majority of them die within two years of admission. But as the current trend toward lay and professional understanding of the needs and capabilities of elderly people increases, more families will want to develop such alternatives to institutionalization as home care.[7]

Institutionalization is harder on older people than almost anyone else. Older people do better mentally and physically in their own homes and in settings familiar to them. The older we grow, the more accustomed we become to certain behavior patterns, and the more our physiology adapts to these patterns. Change is stressful at any age, even when it is voluntary, and it becomes more stressful as we grow older, especially if it is imposed upon us. Home is where the heart is — especially for older people — therefore, we should do all we can to provide home services for those who don't absolutely need hospitalization. At home, the patient can enjoy the warmth, dignity, and privacy inherently lacking in an institution. At home, patients are with family and friends, aided in their daily living and spiritually reinforced by them, and most important, it has been found that they convalesce more rapidly and retain their independence longer in familiar surroundings.

Psychological investigations of aging have found that life satisfaction is an important influence on successful aging and quality of health of the older individual. These studies have found that the environmental setting in which older persons live correlates to their life satisfaction. The more constraints put on individuals, as in an institution, the lower their satisfaction and the worse off they are physically and mentally.[9]

Being able to stay in their own homes, a famliar and stable place, helps not only the physical, but also the psychological well-being of many elderly people. The home is a significant place to many older persons. It is part of their identity, a place where things are familiar and relatively unchanging, and a place in which to maintain a sense of autonomy and control. Most older people have the desire for as much freedom and independence as possible. They fear the loss of contact with family members and loved people, places, and things. Many think of hospitals and nursing homes as "houses of death" from which there is no return. The idea of a personal home is deeply ingrained, and communal living is viewed as a loss of personal liberty and dignity. The institution, therefore, is not the place to send an elderly person, especially just for maintenance or custodial care.[10]

In reality, nursing homes have offered neither maintenance nor custodial care, and in too many ways they have been negligent to their patients. They have deprived human beings of their sense of dignity, and of their sense of hope too. Patients have felt abandoned, discarded and frightened. It is not surprising that those people in nursing homes who retained their sense of identification with society deteriorate rapidly (because the contrast is so great), and that others who deny the reality of their situation retreat to other times and places, when their feelings and their sense of self were more bearable. The psychological cost of institutionalization of the elderly person is becoming a matter of great concern, and now even some hospitals are developing home care programs that address a person's emotional and physical needs.[11]

Home care for the confused elderly can be especially benefical psycholgically. Keeping these people at home provides a normal and familiar environment for them. Familiar surroundings are reassuring and the older person does not need to be separated from family members, friends, possessions, and pets. Problems of these confused people can be averted by reducing the amount of change in their lives. Many of these people can be treated successfully at home because the relatives or friends caring for them are able to adapt to the new problems the confusion creates.[12]

One such success story is told by Judy Henri about her family's deinstitutionalization of her father-in-law, who was diagnosed as having vascular organic brain syndrome. He had been placed in a retirement center in the Midwest, but the family became alarmed at his increased rate of deterioration, passivity, and dependency while he was there, so they decided to bring him home and care for him there. With the love and special attention that he received in a familiar environment, he began to do more for himself, to walk with a livelier gait, and to hum when he was content. The family knew he would not have spontaneously improved to such an extent if they had left him in the institution.[13]

Not all old people want to stay out of institutions. Some elderly people welcome this transition as a freedom from care. Some families are not able to cope psychologically and physically with illnesses in their homes, and the older person may be happier and safer in an institution. But they should at least have the choice.[14]

## Psychological Effects of Home Care on the Dying

The surroundings of a dying person play a major role in the kind of death he or she experiences, and though dying at home may not be for everyone, it is the best choice for most people. Feeling secure is a primary need for people who know they are dying, and one of their biggest fears is that of dying alone, isolated from the people they care about. At home, the patient has fewer adjustments to make and familiar faces, foods, sounds, and smells may restore more vitality than any medical treatment could. At home, the family and patient have control over all aspects of the patient's care, and therefore decisions can be made in the best interest of the patient. This gives both the family and the patient a greater feeling of power and control over a situation they can't do anything about. In a hospital, the family and patient often are made to feel helpless. This causes a great deal of anguish and depression which could be prevented if the family takes care of the patient at home. Dying patients should not be abandoned or isolated from their usual sources of spiritual and emotional support. They need to know that they matter to those close to them. At home, with the family caring for the patient, the patient's feelings of loneliness and isolation are reduced. Being able to communicate and resolve the emotional issues that need to be resolved is a very big factor in the psychological well-being of the dying patient as well as the family. In an institution, with uncomfortable rooms, where hospital apparatus surrounds the high hospital bed and visitors have to look up to the patient from a distance, any meaningul communication is just about impossible. At home, the patient and family can have open discussions in private at any time of the day or night (whenever they feel the need) and can have the discussions in a setting that is comfortable and famliar to them, thus facilitating communication to the fullest. The emotional care that the dying person needs cannot be provided in the hospital by nurses.[15]

## Home Care—The Dying Child

Hospitals have traditionally been the setting for the treatment of children dying with cancer. However, when the treatment that requires hospitalization is no longer being used and the child's cancer is still not under control, the wisdom of continued hospitalization is questionable. It has been a commonly accepted belief that better care and greater control of pain and other symptoms are available in the hospital, but this doesn't take into account the feelings and fears of the child.[16]

Separation of a child from family and home during the process leading to death is traumatic. The hospital, though known for its ability to care for the sick, has never been strong on giving the psychological support the patient needs. Dying children react very strongly to any changes in their environment. The hospital, which promotes this anxiety in the child, would seem the last place to put a dying child for comfort and prolonged care. Many hospitalized children feel that they are being sent to the hospital as punishment for dying.[17]

There are many psychological benefits to the dying child who is cared for at home. The child receives the needed security and love that stem from the home environment.[18] Patients also appear to derive much relief from stress by being at home; they can have their parents close by and be in familiar surroundings, eat the food they are used to, pursue normal activities as much as possible, and have the company of their siblings and pets. The importance of such things for children is too often overlooked.

The pressures of separation, loneliness, isolation, and lack of continuity of care — all inherent to the hospital setting — can be avoided by home care, where families can share the responsibilities of providing special care to the dying child with love and affection in comfortable, familiar surroundings.[19]

## Psychological Benefits and Hazards
## of Home Care on the Family

The effect of home care on the family is a very important issue and one that is connected to its success or failure.

Home care can be psychologically rewarding to the caregivers and the rest of the family, but it can also be an emotional strain. In Anne Davis's study on the disabled adult and the caretaking role in the family, subjects emphasized that the experience and responsibility of taking care of a disabled person provided some family members "with more of a life purpose or meaningfulness, and an opportunity to develop more understanding of the human condition." But before reaching this level, in the early stages of home care, families experienced disorganization, panic, self-blame, rationalization, and overwork. They expressed a tremendous need for support, guidance, and services, which in many instances were not forthcoming except from within the family itself.[20]

Few families are prepared for home care of the seriously ill individual, and the task often can be emotionally wearing. It does, however, offer the interested family a challenge with enormous potential for pleasure and satisfaction. A good, caring doctor and friends, neighbors, and relatives are very important in providing the greatly needed emotional support that will relieve some of the strain on the caregiving familiy.[21]

The key to the success of home care is the primary caregiver. Although caretaking duties are often shared by two or more persons, one individual can usually be identified as the primary caregiver. This caregiver's role usually has both rewards and costs. Among the latter is "role fatigue." When a person is confined to the house all day, day after day, to take care of a disabled person, the stress, isolation, and responsibility can become so great that they adversely affect the caregiver physically and mentally. The result is depression and a feeling of hopelessness. Role fatigue can be avoided if there is a division of labor in both the specific chores of caretaking and the provision of emotional support. Relatives, visiting nurses, or aids can visit the home to take over the caretaking duties for a few hours, freeing the primary caregiver to do what he or she wants. The caregiver needs these frequent respites from the caretaking role in order to keep psychologically fit.

The caregiver, who chooses to care for and is deeply committed to the patient, can derive enormous comfort and satisfaction from the patient's positive responses. Nonetheless, the task of caregiving is complex, and there are many possible sources of stress.[23]

## Psychological Effects of Home Care on the Family of the Dying Patient

Home care for the dying person is, in most cases, good for the family as well as the patient. It gives the family something to do that is concretely helpful to the patient and thus reduces the family's sense of helplessness; it also confronts them unambiguously with the reality of dying. Keeping a terminally ill patient at home provides the family with the opportunity to work through their grieving process and eliminate guilt feelings that naturally occur. "Families who cared for loved ones at home had far less grief to work through than families whose loved one died alone one night at the hospital." Home care provides family members with the privilege of saying good-bye, an act that helps set their minds at ease.[24]

Patricia Kennedy, in her book *Dying at Home with Cancer*, writes about her personal experience with home care and the psychological benefits that come from it.

> In our personal case, my family was very sorry when Dad died, but we did not feel that crippling anguish about his parting others exhibited at the funeral. We knew what he had gone through. We also knew we had diminished his discomfort, serving him during his greatest need.
>
> We had the opportunity to watch Dad accept his own dying. At the end, he was not angry or depressed as he had been earlier. We also shared the peace of acceptance that came as a result of talking with him about his dying and helping make it a successful part of living.[25]

Home care can also be a profound emotional burden with a tremendous amount of stress on the family, but with help from expert counselors, physicians, nurses, and other caregivers trained in hospice care these burdens can be lightened and the experience can become a better one for both the patient and family. As Martin Shephard remarked, helping someone you love to the exit door instead of leaving that job to others can be one of the richest personal experiences in both your life and the life that is ending.[26]

Psychological benefits of home care for the family of the dying child deserve special mention. Not only do the children who are placed in the hospital become more anxious, but the lives of the family members also become more stressful. Because of the structure and regimentation of hospital care, the family can't do much for the dying child without the permission of someone on the hospital staff. Parents have no control over the situation, which makes them feel inadequate and helpless. In the home, the desire to maintain an active role in their child's care and to have constant access to their child is fulfilled. This helps displace the feelings of guilt that frequently follow the death of a child. It has also been found that parents who take care of their child at home return to "normal" sooner after the child's death, and they seem to dwell more on the positive aspects of their child's life than on the bitterness associated with the loss of their child.[27]

The psychological effects of home care on the siblings of the dying child are also very important. If the child dies in the hospital, siblings may believe that the hospital, not the disease, killed their brother or sister. They often have feelings of guilt as well as the fear that the same thing will happen to them. With the child at home, the siblings can participate in caregiving and they can more easily establish the link between illness and death. Studies have found that no great amount of distress or behavioral problems have appeared in the siblings of the children who died at home, and although the loss of a sibling may have a psychological impact on a child whatever the case, it appears that witnessing death does not cause any special adverse reactions.[28]

One of the biggest psychological benefits of home care for the family is the feeling that they did all they could while the patient was alive, so that when the patient dies there is less guilt and it is easier for the family to accept the death and go on with their lives.

The psychological benefits of home care, to most patients, are so great that families and close friends should do all they can to keep their sick, disabled, dying, or elderly family members out of institutional settings and in familiar surroundings whenever possible. Very few people enjoy being in a hospital or any other institutional setting. Most of these institutions are impersonal, dehumanizing, and humiliating places. It is hard for people to be "up" mentally in this type of an environment, and this has a major effect on a person's physical well-being. The mental and physical are so closely intertwined that both have to be treated in order for the patient to recover as quickly as possible, in the case of the sick or injured person, or to feel the best that they can and live as fully as possible, in the case of the disabled, dying, or elderly person. In an institutional setting the staff is usually overworked just taking care of the physical aspects of the patient's illnesses, and they don't have time to get to know the person inside the body. Even if they did have the time to get to know the feelings and needs of the patient, there are so many other environmental constraints in institutions inhibiting the emotional well-being of the patient that the treatment may still not be as effective as it could be in a less routinized, more personal home setting.

Just about any patient who is not in critical condition and in need of hospital equipment and expert physical care could benefit from *good* home care, but too often the home care that the patient receives is not the supporting, loving care that is emotionally uplifting and beneficial to the patient. Caring for someone at home can be very trying, tiring, and emotionally draining for the caregiver and the family. For everyone to get the most out of home care, the caregiver (whether it be a family member, friend, or special nurse) has to be devoted to and care for the patient as a person. If they don't care, the negative aspects will dominate and home care will not help anyone. I have seen cases where families have taken in elderly parents, more out of a sense of obligation and guilt than devotion and caring. They have become resentful toward the patient and this creates an environment that is stressful for everyone involved. This is not good home care and the patient and family would probably be better off if other arrangements were made.

Good home care comes from a loving, patient, and understanding caregiver who gets lots of helping and emotional support from family, friends, physicians, counselors, and other home health care providers and programs that are available. People who are going to take on the responsibility of home care need to be educated on the physical health care needs of the patient. They need to feel confident that they can handle any situation that might arise. They need to be able to have someone to call for help when they need it. Without this education and support the caregiver is scared, stressed, and tense all the time, and it is impossible for home care to be an enjoyable or beneficial situation for anyone.

Getting this needed support and education can be a problem because there are few programs available, and those that exist are often understaffed and underfunded and, therefore, not really brought to the public's attention. This is especially true in smaller towns, where there may be no home health care programs at all. Depending on the circumstances, home care may not be a good choice. It may be too much of a strain on everyone. Maybe as more people begin to realize the benefits of home care, more time and money will be spent on developing and coordinating good home care programs.

Deciding whether to institutionalize a loved family member can be one of the hardest and most emotional times in a family's life. Just having to make this decision can cause a great amount of stress and emotional upheaval in the lives of everyone involved. But if home care programs were made readily available, people educated in the positive aspects of home care for them as well as the patient, and in how to deal with the problems that may arise, maybe they wouldn't see home care as such a burden. Maybe fewer people would have to face the decision of whether to institutionalize the family member. Home care would just seem the natural thing to do.

# 5

# THE ECONOMICS
# OF HOME CARE

Home care was the original form of medical care, long before hospitals existed. When hospitals did appear on the
scene, they were frequently regarded as "death houses," and the sick
were really better off remaining at home. Of course, the hospitals
eventually did succeed in its own right as an institution where certain
diseases were treated effectively. Today, with the economic situation
being what it is, along with intense government pressure to curb rising health care costs, we may have gone full circle. The home is once
again a viable alternative to care in an institution.

Debate over potential savings of home health care as opposed to
hospitalization has gone on for years. Much of the comparison has
centered on the belief that if health service is provided in the home
instead of an institution, savings will be realized from decreased admissions, earlier discharges, and reduced capital construction costs
for new inpatient facilities. Critics point out that there might be a
cost savings for patients with low levels of impairment, but the savings
tend to disappear when the severely impaired are cared for at home.[1]
They go on to claim that increased availability of home health care
may increase the total costs of health care by increased overall utilization.

Many of these studies, however, were done when home care was
first being evaluated as a health care alternative.[2] Since there was
relatively little funding for home health care, the studies can hardly
be considered representative of its potential. Also, the medical profession has always tried to maintain the status quo, particularly when
a perceived threat to economic enrichment is involved. Witness the

objection by the AMA to insurance coverage at its inception, and also to health maintenance organizations in the early 1970s.

With all the discussion of health care using the terms "cost benefit" and "cost effectiveness," these terms need to be defined. In cost-benefit analysis, the cost of a health expenditure is compared with estimates of the monetary value of benefits that are realized as a result. Cost-effectiveness analysis — a narrower application of cost-benefit analysis — compares the cost of alternative ways of achieving a similar set of results.[3] The cases herein will compare home health services and the institutional alternative.

Costs of home health care are dependent on several variables, including patient impairment levels, quality of care, type of care rendered, available family support, and proper utilization levels. It is felt that many of the studies indicating cost benefits and lack of cost benefits for home care neglect the fact that they are isolated studies. When home care is incorporated as a "total system," it could ultimately prove to be cost effective.

Other benefits of home care besides potential cost savings include:

1. Homebound people can be taught to live relatively independent status.

2. Efficiency of the practicing physician can be increased by expanding the team approach.

3. The physician can care for a greater number of patients through a home care program, because he does not have to assemble and coordinate individually the services needed for patients in their home settings.

4. Home care staff can readily interpret medical orders, explain treatment regimens, and offer reassurance and support.

5. Home care staff can identify day-to-day problems, and thereby help to reduce the possibility of emergency situations arising.[4]

Some of the different aspects of home health care financing to be examined include the question of why something that has been around so long has seen such little development. Also, what Medicare changes have eased home health care financing? Also to be discussed are home care economics in terminal illness, treating the elderly, home parenteral (intravenous) nutrition, dialysis at home, home hospice care, respiratory therapists and home care, and an example of hospital-based home care. Finally, we will look at why home care involvement is advantageous to hospitals and make some recommendations on how to improve home health care financing.

Home health care can be defined as "a combination of health care and social services rendered to individuals and families in their homes or other community settings. Medical needs first are established by a physician, and a plan of care is developed. Subsequent professional care received in the home can include skilled nursing; physician care; dietary advice; occupational, physical, recreational, and speech therapy; and laboratory services. Other services are home delivered meals, companionship, and patient and family education."[5]

There are those who have described home health care as an "eighteen-year old baby."[6] This description seems more than appropriate when one considers that it has been around for some time, although placed on the "back burner" in terms of development. Low priority for home health care advancement by policy makers has led to inhibition of progress.

Home care was born in the mid-1960s when Congress passed the Medicare "conditions of participation" for home health agencies. Little legislation of significance was passed to help further progress until the lifting of the ban on home care without state licensure. Congress also passed a law offering three-year Medicaid-funded demonstration projects to states providing home- and community-based care. As of November 1982, thirty-two states had filed for participation. In January 1983, President Reagan signed the Orphan Drug Act, which authorized $5 million in loans and grants to proprietary and nonprofit agencies to expand home health service in underserved rural and urban areas during fiscal years 1983 and 1984.

Why has the federal government suddenly taken such a big interest in home health care? The bottom line is simply the dollars to be saved and the demographics of the situation. Lawmakers realized that health care costs, particularly for the elderly, are likely to continue to spiral unless drastic measures are taken. Home care is proving itself a cost-effective alternative. With funds diminishing and the aged population on the rise, an alternative to the high cost of institutional care is necessary.

When looking objectively at the situation from a humanitarian point of view, few elderly people want to go to a nursing home. Anything reasonable that will help them maintain their independence and quality of life is preferable to an institution. Peoria, Illinois, is one of the few places that has had a licensed home health program since 1966.[7] The program has grown tremendously since its inception. The 1,215 home visits in 1966 had almost tripled to 3,054 by 1975. By 1982, the figure rose to 13,345. Part of this large growth was attributable to the fact that, since 1976, the program has had a nurse coordinator who assists with hospital discharge planning. Doctor referrals have also contributed to increased use of the program. Something as simple as awareness of the services available on the part of physicians has helped. Also, family practice residents have been taken on home visits, which has increased physician awareness.

Some of the advantages of home health services have been cited by Phillip Sellers, a Hendersonville, North Carolina, internist.[8] Besides the cheaper cost as compared to institutional care, he mentions that patients can avoid such hospital hazards as confusion, infection, disorientation, falls, personality conflicts, noise, and anxiety. Sellers mentions, however, that areas with home health agencies have a monopoly on care. He claims that Medicare will not reimburse for his nurse or other paramedical personnel making a home visit, but it will pay for an agency nurse. Sellers goes on to say that Medicare will pay him $21.50 for a routine house call, and a home health agency nurse $40. Frequently doctors in this program do not see patients for long periods of time, and this leads to poor medical practice.

In 1981, Senator Orrin Hatch (R-Utah), chairman of the Senate Labor and Human Resources Committee, had the General Accounting Office (GAO) look into whether or not expanding home care would result in cost reduction. The GAO concluded that although home care increased the longevity and life satisfaction of the elderly, it did not decrease nursing home utilization. The GAO saw expanding home care services as more of an addition to, and not a substitute for, institutional care. The GAO went on to say, however, that were eligibility for home health services tightly controlled for a specific population, a cost savings could be realized.

Several changes occurred in Medicare home health care financing as of July 1, 1981, that have made receiving finances under Part A easier, as well as reducing the cost under Medicare, Part B. These include:

1. The elimination of the three-day prehospitalization requirement in Part A.

2. Requiring care given to be skilled care, rather than the previously required continuation of acute hospital care (also Part A).

3. Lifting the one-hundred-visit-per-year limit to permit unlimited visits when medically justified (Parts A and B).

4. Elimination of the $60 deductible in Part B.[9]

Blue Cross studies conducted in Pennsylvania, New York, Colorado, and Oregon have indicated a decrease in the number of hospital days when home health care was an intensive, short-term nursing extension of acute care. The use of home care to replace institutional care of chronically impaired patients, however, has questionable cost-effectiveness. Studies done in North Carolina and Minnesota indicate that for 91 percent of patients in nursing homes any other type of care was economically infeasible. This particular study was deceptive in that it failed to measure social factors. (e.g. willingness of the family to care for the patient upon leaving the institution). It can also be assumed, therefore, that although home care has many economic advantages over institutional care, there are situations when the services required for the patient make it more expensive.

Why aren't home health care services more popular? Federal, state, and local governments are all aware that home services are not coordinated effectively. There are three separate entities in the Department of Health and Human Services that are responsible for handling home-related health services. These agencies include the Public Health Service, the Office of Long Term Care, and the Administration on Aging, all of which apparently function independently. In Pennsylvania, for example, there are three more independent state agencies. These agencies have 117 local home health agencies under their jurisdiction. Congress helped to ease the Medicare/Medicaid reimbursement for home care when it passed Public Law 96-499, which waived the requirement that for-profit home health agencies must be licensed by the state they are in before receiving Medicare or Medicaid funds.

As mentioned, prior to the twentieth century, hospitals were places where people went to die. Although the 1900s saw the rise of treatment and cure, ironically, hospitals are again popular places for people to die. Death has been institutionalized, just as education, birth, and other aspects of life. And as increased resources have gone to many other medical concerns, so too have they risen for care of the dying patient. But there has been a direct correlation between increased funds for care of the dying and the degree of dissatisfaction for patient and family. Reasons for this include unfamiliar surroundings to the patient and separation from the support and comfort of the family.[10]

With these factors in mind, Bernard Bloom and Priscilla Kissick performed a study on patients with two weeks to live and compared charges generated for home care with those for patients spending a similar period in a hospital.[11] Family members kept detailed records of costs incurred, as well as family and patient reaction to the caring process. Hospital accounting departments provided itemization of charges for inpatients with terminal disease.

The results were astoundingly in favor of home care. Charges for hospital care were ten and a half times greater than the home counterpart. The mean charge for patients dying at home for the final two weeks was $586, with a range of from $137 to $1,162. The cost for those dying in a hospital had a mean of $6,180, with a range of from $3,333 to $11,645. The per diem home care charge was $42, compared with $441 for hospital care. It must be noted that the care given in the hospitals in the study was complex and expensive, and probably would have been significantly less if provided by a community hospital.[12]

The study by Bloom and Kissick indicates the great cost-effectiveness of home care for the patient with two weeks to live, when compared with comparable care in a hospital. Although the topic of this chapter is the economics of home care, some mention must be made here of other factors. The great disparity in the charges necessitates a look at whether or not the terminal patient is better off at home than in an institution. Diaries provided by family members indicate that besides cost savings, the experience of providing care for a dying loved one was a worthwhile, satisfying experience.[13] Most were able to provide the necessary care with little professional assistance.

With death being a foregone conclusion for all the patients in the study, one must ask why so much was spent for the hospital inpatients on items such as X-rays, blood transfusions, and respiratory therapy. Certainly pain relief and comfort could be provided a terminal patient without maximizing charges during their final days. By dealing with individual symptoms instead of the inevitable outcome for the patient medical practitioners are avoiding the true nature of their patient's needs. Even worse, they apparently are charging the patient and the insurance company as much as possible before the patient dies. With the cost difference and other benefits of home care for the terminal patient, as compared with the intensive services and high expense of treating the terminally ill in hospitals, current government policy on these alternatives must be examined if we are serious about cost containment. The outcome in either case is the same.

Obviously, if care can be provided for an elderly individual at home, a savings would be realized. Not only are there monetary advantages, but also social benefits and the fostering of independence. Unfortunately, the elderly are often institutionalized because there are no available home care or community support services. It should be noted that Medicaid spending for nursing homes totaled $5.6 billion in 1977.[14] Also, care in skilled nursing facilities is a mandated basic Medicaid service for all individuals over twenty-one years of age; and in nineteen states, nursing homes account for the bulk of Medicaid expenditures. But Medicaid is not the only source of funding for long-term care of the elderly; Medicare, veterans benefits, Supplemental Security Income, social service, and various state and local programs contribute heavily.

With all this in mind, noninstitutionalized care for the elderly certainly has to be the desirable cost-containing alternative. It is not so easy, however, as many of the elderly are poor and have no spouse or children to assist them. Also, families either refuse to or cannot assist elderly individuals whether due to distance, living facilities, family structures, or financial limitations. Therefore, if no social support is forthcoming from family or friends, a nursing home is the grim alternative. With the percentage of elderly expected to increase dramatically between now and the year 2000, demands on long-term care facilities will also increase and the home care alternative must be developed to relieve society of some of the economic burden.

It is estimated that three hundred thousand elderly in the United States are inappropriately placed in nursing homes. Conservative estimates for home care place the cost at about $400 per month versus $700 per month and up for institutionalized care.[15] The figures indicate potential cost reductions of upwards of $1 billion per year. This figure does not include savings derived from not having to expand facilities. Of course there are sociological and psychological benefits to the home care alternatives for which a dollar value cannot be assigned.

In studies, Dunlop found that increases in home care were associated with decreases in nursing homes and related facilities. While investigating 245 patients in a New York City program for the home-bound aged, Brickner reported that after two years 23 patients had improved to the extent that they were no longer homebound, 116 remained stabilized under the program's continuing care, and 40 patients were institutionalized in hospitals or nursing homes. The clinical judgment was that without the program 85 of the patients would have received institutionalized care, 25 would have needed but not have received institutionalized care, and 25 would have died.[16]

The implication is, therefore, that many of the elderly are institutionalized more frequently and earlier than is actually necessary. Also a large cost savings could be realized to society if older people were not institutionalized until greatly impaired. It is ironic that 17 percent of those sixty-five or over fall into the "greatly impaired" category and one-third of them are in institutions.[17]

Medicare and Medicaid are the driving forces in formation and implementation of long-term care policies for government. The lack of priority given to home health care is apparent when one notes that Medicare and Medicaid spend only $356 million for home health care as compared to $5.6 billion for institutional care. Why not pay nurses to provide the same level of care in the home of the patient? The nursing home could manage the patient's case without having the patient physically reside in the facility, and at least some savings (i.e., building and maintenance) would be realized.

A program similar to this is the "nursing home without walls" instituted in New York in 1978.[18] Besides basic nursing, the program provides such services as home health aides; physical, occupational, respiratory, and speech therapists; nutrutional services; homemaker and housekeeper services; and medical supplies and appliances. There is, of course, a physician who periodically monitors patient progress, as would be the case in an institution. The savings in this program for New York were 25 percent or $11.8 million.

Gerontologist Andrew Dibner has developed a unique new home monitoring system for the elderly known as "Lifeline."[19] With this system disabled persons wear an electronic device that functions for twenty-four hours. Then the patient must reset the timer, which signals to the Lifeline system the patient's well-being. Should the timer not be reset, a buzzer and light flash on the home unit, and the emergency station is automatically called. In the event an emergency is signaled, a cental operator telephones the user, who can reset the monitor if it is a false alarm. Should the patient not answer when an emergency is signaled, the Lifeline operator has a list of people to call (neighbors, relatives) who will attend to the patient. The operator can send a signal back to the patient that turns off the alarm on the monitor, notifying him or her that help is on the way.

The Lifeline system was evaluated in the Boston-Cambridge area using medically vulnerable or functionally impaired elderly. Thirty percent of the sample members were over eighty years old, with an overall mean of seventy-five years. It was believed prior to the study that there would be a cost benefit to the program as compared to traditional long-term care options. Benefits attributable to Lifeline included direct savings from reduction of health facility and community service use, as well as nonmarket or intangible benefits. The benefit/ cost ratio was the greatest for those "severely functionally impaired, but not socially isolated" and either "moderately functionally impaired" or "medically vulnerable." Lifeline results indicated that fewer medical and social support resources, as well as fewer acute hospital and nursing home days were used by participants than those in control groups. Overall economic value of the reduced medical and social support service utilization was estimated at $62,484, yeilding a benefit/cost ratio of 1.87.

Many patients, for one reason or another, must be on parenteral (intravenous) nutritional programs. Some of the more common diseases that force dependence on this form of nutrition include Crohn's Disease and Short Bowel Syndrome. Jane I. Brakebill et al. performed a study at the University of Washington in Seattle to compare costs of home parenteral nutrition versus those generated when hospitalizing for the procedure.[20] The patients in the study were selected from a group of fifty-five already active in a home parenteral nutrition program (HPN). Cost items identified included supplies, personnel, freight, equipment, miscellaneous and indirect costs. The charges for HPN patients also include laboratory tests and clinic visits. Charges for inpatients were identified in a similar manner and included the standard daily hospital charge.

Results of the study were astoundingly in favor of HPN as a cost-effective alternative. The average charge per infusion day for HPN patients was $48 versus $205 for the same procedure in a hospital. Savings generated per patient, therefore, were $157, or a difference of 76 percent. When multiplying that figure times the average number of infusion days per year (209), the total savings per patient comes to $32,915. Some important points to note about the study are that the patients were taught to mix their own solutions, and 90 percent of those in the study were women. (Women usually do not have as great a nutritional requirement as men.) Both of these factors resulted in cost savings, but even without them, home parenteral nutrition represents a genuine cost savings.

It is well documented that since the advent of hemodialysis in 1960, survival rates for patients with end-stage kidney disease have increased. Although most patients on home dialysis have or require the assistance of a spouse or relative, there are a few who can perform it on their own at home. By and large, though, dialysis patients need the assistance of another person. Unfortunately, many patients suitable for home dialysis have no relative to assist them or have medical complications that preclude treatment of this type. A study performed in Canada found that through the use of paid dialysis helpers visiting either the home or a limited-care facility, a substantial savings could be realized over the alternative, inpatient dialysis. Not only was the dollars savings per patient considerable ($10,000 to $15,000), but there were also benefits in the form of stress reduction for the family and patient just by being in the home rather than in an institution. Home care is more cost-effective than hospital care for the routine dialysis patient with a family assistant, and it can also be cost-effective in almost all but acute cases when a trained professional can visit the patient at home.[21]

The home-care hospice alternative is another viable alternative to institutionalization. It provides many of the same services within the four walls of the patient's home and shows a cost savings. Hospice of Columbus (HOC) in Columbus, Ohio, conducted a study evaluating home hospice care in terms of evaluations of families who used the care and the cost of services rendered.[22]

Cancer patients accepted into the HOC program needed the support of a physician who would assume responsibility for medical followup and nursing management at home. The typical patient had to be eighteen years old, live in the metropolitan area of Columbus, and have a remaining life span estimated at two days to six months. Family and patient had to be aware of the diagnosis and prognosis and agree to the concept of providing merely supportive care. One person in the family was designated as primary caregiver and acted as a link to the hospice staff. In most cases, this role was filled by the spouse, with an adult child being the second most common caregiver.

Results of the study compared costs to those generated in the local community for a hospital or nursing home alternative. The hospital charges were $126 per day or $5,292 for forty-two days, which was the mean life span of patients in the study. For skilled care at a nursing home, typical charges were $50 per day or $2,100 for the forty-two day period. Care provided by HOC at home was only slightly less than $2,000 for the forty-two day period, indicating only a mild economic advantage for home hospice care over the institutional alternatives. One must remember, however, that other benefits such as patient preference, family involvement, and avoidance of using a facility that could be used by a more needy patient are not easily quantified in dollars and cents.

As with many other disciplines in the allied health field, the situation is a little different for respiratory-care specialists seeking to perform care at home as a cost-effective alternative. Joseph Califano's statement in May 1977 that "of 700,000 patients in acute care hospitals, 100,000 of them could be better treated at home" comes across to respiratory therapists (RTs) as little more than the government's convoluted logic. On the one hand, the government urges increased home care as a cost-saving measure, yet Medicare will only pay for in-hospital treatments and not the same therapy at home. And of course, the majority of respiratory-therapy patients are elderly people who are dependent upon Medicare. The lack of recognition has stifled growth of this home-care service. RTs have gone so far as to give treatments at home for free, which naturally generates hostility.

Part of the irony is that when a typical respiratory patient is admitted with little more than mild exacerbation of a lung problem, he not only accrues charges for respiratory treatments, but also the room charge and other charges for items he may have at home anyway, but are considerably marked up in price by the hospital (aspirin, bronchodilators). Since many of those with mild exacerbation of lung disease cannot get a trained professional reimbursed for coming to their home and treating their acute process when it is mild, patients must wait until their condition is so poor as to justify inpatient status to receive the therapy they need. This results in charges for admission (which could possibly have been avoided through proper home therapy by a trained professional), as well as patients who are much sicker than they would have been, were the acute process checked earlier by home care. Another irony is Medicare's willingness to reimburse for rental charges on respiratory equipment, but not for any of the trained service that goes along with the devices. Essentially, Medicare is acknowledging the expertise of the machine and not the professional. To complicate the situation further, Medicare does not fully reimburse for the equipment.

Since respiratory therapists are trained professionals accredited by the National Board of Registered Therapists, it would be inappropriate to drop a machine off on a patient's doorstep and drive off. In fact, many patients do not even require a machine to get the therapy they need. Procedures such as postural drainage and percussion to clear phlegm from the lungs are performed by a trained professional using his or her hands, not machinery. Also provided is education of the patient and family, which goes a lot farther than the temporary symptomatic relief achieved with the aid of a machine. To third-party reimbursement organizations (Blue Cross, Blue Shield, Medicaid, private insurers), these types of treatments are apparently meaningless. There is evidence that were the third parties to reimburse therapists for home care, they would realize significant savings. South Hills Health Service in Pittsburgh, Pennsylvania,[23] conducted a study to determine costs of hospitalization versus home care, using one hundred home care patients who previously had been hospitalized. Total cost for in-hospital services was estimated at $120,000. Respiratory therapists then visited the same patients at home on a monthly basis and initially found there to be a 50 percent average decrease in charges. After paperwork and other charges were figured, the study concluded savings to be 36 percent.

Another example was a study done by Home Services Division in Minneapolis, Minnesota.[24] There, an infant at home was provided with low-flow oxygen to a head box and periodically received other respiratory services, such as suctioning. After a year available estimates were that charges for the same support in a hospital would have been $176,000, whereas it cost $2,400 to receive the therapy at home by a trained professional with equipment. Of course, the $176,000 figure includes all those charges not respiratory related that would be generated as an inpatient. The savings of about $173,000 to the third-party reimbursement agency is dramatic.

Senate Bill 2009 is an attempt to clear away some of the inequities of home care reimbursement. Although respiratory care is not specifically mentioned, the bill states that "Medicare should cover all levels of home care for a patient, depending on his assessed need." Heretofore Medicare has not had reimbursement policies for home respiratory care due to its low priority on Medicare's list of services. As the incidence of emphysema and other chronic lung conditions has increased, however, Medicare's priorities may start to change. With the goal of SB2009 being to keep people out of institutions, recognition of the value of home respiratory care could prove very cost-effective. The care would be formulated by a physician and done by a respiratory therapist, and there would be periodic reports by the doctor to Medicare to justify continued need for home therapy. Other third-party reimbursers would likely fall in line behind Medicare once the precedent is set.

Many of the nearly half a million people in Tucson are victims of cardiopulmonary disease; the warm, dry climate attracts those with breathing difficulties. As recently as 1970, St. Joseph's Hospital of Tucson examined the home care situation locally and found no agency providing this form of care.[25] The routine of a medical supply company sending over a truck driver to drop off a device was typical. Patients were also frequently hospitalized, not out of medical necessity, but because it was the only way insurance paid for their care. Since there was little in the way of patient education following an acute episode, patients were frequently rehospitalized soon after. St. Joseph's began a home therapy program treating a wide variety of lung diseases, including emphysema, bronchitis, asthma, and bronchiectasis. It also established a "Better Breathing Club" whose function was to educate patients and families as to basic lifestyle changes that would result in more healthy time for the respiratory patient. All treatment modes common to respiratory therapy were incorporated, with an emphasis on nonmechanical means (i.e., no machines) whenever possible. A physician followed patient progress and had input into the appropriate therapy.

The study followed 44 patients over a 29-month period. In the year prior to the home care program, the 44 patients were admitted to St. Joseph's 151 times. During the 29-month period, the same group was hospitalized 93 times. Previous hospitalizations averaged 17 days, whereas after home care they averaged 15 days.

A hospital-based home care program (HHC) does exist, and it

makes use of the institution's potential for providing effective care at home as well as on an inpatient basis.[26] Since the program is labor-intensive, startup costs are minimal. In 1974, Blue Cross established guidelines for HHC plans if reimbursement were to be applied for. The guidelines included an "intensive" category of HHC benefits, which requires professional coordination of health care services, central administration of those services, and active medical and nursing management of patient care; "intermediate" benefits, which are less concentrated and usually focus on a single service or combination of nursing and therapeutic services; and a "basic" category, which involves the minimum services needed to maintain a patient's health and well-being. Emphasis by Blue Cross is on use of the intermediate and intensive categories, as it is felt that these areas show the greatest potential for containing health care costs. The HHC plans provide physical therapy, nurse home visits, respiratory therapy, occupational therapy, prescription services, prosthetic devices, medical and surgical supplies, and ambulance and outpatient services. Going along with the intensive and intermediate category emphasis, the plans do not provide nutritional guidance, homemaker services, or home health aides.

Studies done on HHC programs in Philadelphia between 1962 and 1970 showed a savings of $330 per case, and in Michigan during the same period, $519 to $917 per case. Both figures are from the intensive and intermediate categories. The HHC case is an excellent example of hospital involvement saving health dollars, as well as cost containment if the hospital does not overinvolve itself (e.g., homemaker services).

As mentioned before, there is an increasingly finite amount of resources available in this country for health care. With a national inflation average of about 5 percent, the health care industry simply cannot continue raising costs at a rate of almost 16 percent. The federal government began attempts at cost containment during the Carter administration; they were subsequently stifled by the AMA's lobbying organization, AMPAC. The enactment of the Tax Equity and Fiscal Responsibility Act of 1982, however, imposed a three-year, 7.9 percent cap on hospital expense increases.[27] Many believe this is a forerunner of even more restrictive legislation on expenses to come. With all this in mind, the health care industry needs to have new strategies not only for insuring our nation's hospitals, but also for providing quality care for patients. Home care can provide opportunities to meet both these needs.

One may ask, what does a hospital stand to gain by encouraging patients not to use their facilities? When viewed in light of the dwindling amount of resources available for home care, it is easy to see that what exists must be used cost-effectively for maximum patient benefits. It is obvious that decreased levels of care within a hospital setting result in decreased costs for that institution. Telemetry step-down units to complement cardiovascular intensive care are examples of this. Miami Valley Hospital has four levels of care in their regional dialysis center: inpatient dialysis, outpatient staff supported, outpatient, and home dialysis. Each case has diminishing costs as the level of care decreases. Home care, therefore, is merely an extension of this cost-reduction principle.

There are other financial advantages for hospitals in containing costs through increased use of home care. In states such as New York, hospitals are reimbursed only at cost, whereas home health services are fully reimbursed. Depending on the level of participation by a hospital in this case, revenues can be enhanced considerably. Recent legislation in the state of Washington has offered more financial advantages for hospitals willing to contain costs. Hospitals that exceed the 7.9 percent federal cap on expense increases will be penalized seventy-five cents on every dollar they go over the limit. Hospitals remaining under the cap will receive a bonus of 50 percent of savings realized. The home health care advantage of reduced length of hospital stay is a big part of this strategy.

Not to be forgotten in this discussion of financial restrictions on hospitals is Medicare reimbursement. In October 1983, Richard Schweiker, secretary of Health and Human Services, went on record as supporting even more restrictive limitations on Medicare reimbursement. Schweiker's proposal would pay all hospitals the same amount, fixed in advance, for treating any patient with a particular diagnosis. This concept, referred to as diagnosis-related groups (DRGs), would pay every hospital in the United States the same predetermined rate for a tonsillectomy, appendectomy, heart attack, or any other of 467 disease categories. There would be only minor allowances for geographical variances in hospital costs and salaries. Schweiker contends that DRGs provide incentive for hospitals to be more efficient because they could pocket any savings remaining under the fixed payment. For example, if the predetermined rate were $3,300 for a ten-day stay, but the patient could safely be discharged after nine days, the hospital would see a savings of $300. When spread over a number of admissions, savings could be appreciable.

Another financial advantage to the hospital participating in home health care is the potential of freeing up beds needed for those with more serious illness. Some areas in the Sun Belt have a premium on hospital beds, and it is important that a heart attack or severe trauma victim not be denied a bed that is occupied by a marginally ill patient. Also, studies have shown that the highest revenues are generated the first several days of a hospital stay, when most of the testing and treatment is going on.[28] If home care is considered an alternative as soon as the patient is out of danger, considerable cost savings could be realized.

Finally, a financial incentive for hospitals involved in home care can come from drawing on hospital resources. Much of the equipment needed for home health services, such as walkers, dressings, catheters, and syringes, are already part of hospital inventory. The hospital need not worry about constructing facilities, and they also have vast human resources available that would prove useful. There could be flexibility in shifting staff between hospital and home care, which might prove to be a more cost-effective use of personnel, particularly when patient census is low.

Medicare, Medicaid, Blue Cross, and Blue Shield cannot reasonably be expected to pick up all the financial slack necessary to cause home care services in America to grow. Just as HMOs (prepaid care) are taking a bigger portion of health care services from hospitals (fee for service care), so also must there be an element to home care that is an alternative to traditional payment mechanisms. There are several ways this can be facilitated.[29]

The first method is by reduced dependence on government funding. With the current mood of legislators being to trim expenses wherever possible, rising health care costs are a prime target. The Reagan administration philosophy is to reduce government involvement when possible, in favor of the private sector. Home health care in the United States is still in its infancy, and therefore provides fertile ground for the private sector (e.g., insurance companies) to increase their financial interest and work to expand services.

Another alternative to traditional payment mechanisms is through increased contractual services. In many areas of government and in the private sector, contracting out services to private agencies has proven to have cost benefits. It enables a more stable and predictable cash flow for agency budgeting. Also, by contracting services only during the time period necessary, an agency can avoid the "down time" experienced when demand for services is relatively low.

Developing standards for home health agencies is the third method by which they can be improved. Like all relatively new and blossoming markets, home health care is susceptible to those who seek to take financial advantage of the unsuspecting consumer and not provide the type of service the patient needs or is paying for. Here, the American Public Health Association, among other organizations, can become involved in setting standards.

Finally, home health care services need to enlist the help of external grant support. Relatively few people outside of the health care industry and users of the service are aware of home health care. Once it is established as an institution in American life — just as the hospital is now — it will be able to enjoy the same type of grant money hospitals receive from time to time. Undoubtedly, great potential for financial savings and benefit for health care lie in the home industry. It will take responsible planning and development to meet the health needs of society in a cost-efficient manner.

# 6

# THE MAKING OF A
# HOME HEALTH AGENCY

As noted earlier, in 1976 the Boston Dispensary organized this country's first formalized home health agency (HHA). Because the cost of hospitalization for the indigent was so great, the dispensary geared its services toward this group.

The cost of hospitalization and health care today not only puts a burden on the poor, but on the elderly as well. Total U.S. health care expenditures increased $244.9 billion from 1965 to 1981. In 1965, the percentage of federal public funds going toward health care was 25.9; and in 1981, this figure grew to 42.7. Furthermore, hospital care as a percentage of gross national product grew from 33.3 to 41.1 in 1981.

Home health care is a viable solution to the problem of rising health care costs.

The home health care recipient ranges from the newborn to those over one hundred. However, the median age is sixty-nine and the middle 50 percent fall between fifty-nine and seventy-nine.[1] Because the aging constitute the overwhelming majority of the home health care consumers, the prospective supplier of home health care services, for profit if nothing else, would want to focus on this particular group of our society. Further incentives to lure the prospective supplier of home health care to focus on the aging are found in Medicare reimbursement practice. At first, this might sound contradictory, since the goal is to bring down health care expenditures. However, when the cost of home care is compared to the cost of hospitalization, the latter far outweighs the former.

Although similar, Medicare hospital and Medicare medical insurance differ in their reimbursement guidelines for home health care. Medicare hospital insurance reimburses for home health care if all six of the following conditions are met:

• you were in a qualified hospital for at least three days in a row (the day of discharge does not count)
• the home health care is for further treatment of a medical condition that was treated during a hospital stay or covered skilled nursing stay
• you need part-time skilled nursing care of physical or speech therapy
• you are confined to your home (a facility that mainly provides skilled nursing or rehabilitation services cannot be considered your home)
• a doctor prescribes home health care and sets up a home health plan for you within fourteen days of your most recent discharge from a hospital or participating skilled nursing facility
• the home health agency providing services is participating in Medicare

For reimbursement under Medicare medical insurance, the third, fourth, fifth, and sixth conditions must all be met.[2]

If home health care entails both economic and psychological benefits, why has it not caught on? Clair E. Ryder, M.D., director of Ambulatory Care Community Health, HEW, suggests some reasons.[3]

First, home health care is new and different. As one sees with our federal Congress and health care reforms (e.g., Medicare, Medicaid), we as a society tend to move in small increments rather than in a rational, comprehensive way.

Another, more important reason home health care has not caught on involves physicians' attitudes. Physicians believe, according to Dr. Ryder, that if their patients are at home, they are going to have to expend more of their own time traveling around. "Actually it has been shown repeatedly that the reverse is true. There is documented evidence to indicate that the physician's time can be saved because of additional professional hands, eyes, and ears already caring for the patient in his own home."[4] The issue boils down to economic or income maintenance. Patients who are not in the hospital are basically out of the hands of the physician and, hence, out of economic reach of the physician. A physician is the only individual who can recommend a person for home health care, that is, if that person wants Medicare to pick up the bill. The physician's rule extends over the entire health care industry, but their influence specifically on home health care needs to be examined.

## The Accreditation Process

The prospective supplier of home health care should consider accreditation by the National League for Nursing (NLN) and the American Public Health Association (APHA). Although accreditation is optional, there is a definite advantage: Medicare, Blue Cross, and private health insurers will only reimburse if the home health care provider is accredited.

Quality is usually the justification for any type of accreditation, certification, or licensing. Accreditation, however, can be carried to extremes in the name of quality or income maintenance (e.g., plumbers, barbers). Given the increasing amount of fraud related to home health care, though, accreditation seems justified. The NLN-APHA state their purposes for accreditation as follows:

• to stimulate the continuous improvement of community health services
• to promote the coordination and integration of quality health care by all disciplines in community health agencies
• to encourage experimentation and innovation in providing services that meet the standards of accreditation
• to foster the best possible use of available health manpower
• to establish among community agencies a climate of self-study and self-evaluation using accepted criteria
• to help the consumer identify those community services that have met nationally accepted standards
• to guide potential staff to agencies that have indicated a concern for rendering high-quality services
• to aid educational programs in the selection of field laboratories for student learning[5]

Furthermore, before prospective suppliers of home health care apply for accreditation, they must first see if they are eligible. All of the following conditions must be met: the agency has legal authorization to operate, the service has been in continuous operation for at least one year, all service components in a single agency are to be included in the accreditation, the agency has five or more full-time nurses on the staff, and payment for accreditation fees has been authorized.[6]

According to the NLN-APHA, the definition for a home health care agency, for accreditation purposes, is as follows: an organization that basically provides multidisciplinary health care on a family-centered basis to the sick, disabled, or injured in the place of residence; it may also provide programs in addition to care of the sick. Accreditation is based on the agency's self-study report and on the report of the on-site visit by a team of visitors. This self-study report contains eight sections: identifying information (form obtained from NLN), summary positions (form obtained from NLN), organization and administration, program, staff, future plans, an appendix, and any additional materials requested. The specific criteria for each of the above categories will now be discussed in detail.

## Organizational and Administration Criteria

1. The agency is legally authorized and has a governing body responsible for its operation.

2. Consumers of service and representatives of the broad community participate in agency affairs through heterogeneous, active citizen groups. Participation may be through governing board, advisory committees, and/or other arrangements.

3. Administrative responsibilities and relationships are established and clearly defined.

4. The governing body delegates to an individual the authority and responsibility for overall agency administration. The governing body delegates to a qualified health professional from a profession involved in implementing the agency's programs, the authority and responsibility to:

    a. plan, administer, and coordinate the services and program of the agency;

    b. participate in the deliberation and decisions made on policies guiding services and program.

5. Administrative policy and management activities assure effective implementation of the program.

6. The agency is coordinated with other community health facilities and services. It cooperates with organized groups and takes initiative in promoting needed community action.

7. The agency conducts or participates in a planned evaluation of its organization and administration. All health disciplines providing service and other agency staff are involved in this evaluation process.

## Program Criteria

1. The skill, knowledge, and ability of a variety of community groups and individuals, as well as those responsible for implementing the agency's services, are utilized in an ongoing assessment of current health needs and planning agency services to meet these needs.

2. Programs are established, reviewed, and modified to keep pace with current health needs. The agency has specific objectives for each program offered.

3. The agency has priorities for each program and for each service related to agency purpose and community need.

4. The agency has written policies.

5. Service records are maintained for planning and improving all services to individuals, families, and groups.

6. Conferences of workers providing services to a patient/family are held. A professional nurse has the responsibility for coordinating the agency plan for patient care.

7. The agency has an established mechanism for ongoing review of the quality of service rendered by each discipline.

8. The agency has established procedures for program evaluation.

9. If appropriate and feasible, the agency accepts responsibility for participation in the education of health personnel.

## Staff Criteria

1. Health care services are directed and/or coordinated by a health professional from a discipline providing agency service.

2. For all professional personnel, the agency provides ongoing supervision, peer review, or consultation by a qualified co-professional.

**3.** The service staff includes professional personnel who meet the standards for employment of their respective professional organizations.

**4.** Supportive assistance to the service staff is provided by business and office personnel.

**5.** Agency consultants may serve as liaison persons with their co-professionals in other community agencies.

**6.** Personnel policies delineate the conditions of employment and the respective obligations between the employer and employee for all salaried, hourly, or contract personnel. The agency is an equal opportunity employer and has a program of affirmative action.

**7.** Assignment of responsibility provides for appropriate utilization of every employee.

**8.** Each employee has ongoing professional or technical supervision to promote individual development and performance.

**9.** The agency provides orientation and in-service education for each discipline and each classification of worker.

**10.** Staff patterns, policies, and practices are evaluated, in relation to fulfilling the purpose of the agency.

### Future Plans Criteria

Upon completion and submission of the agency's self-study report, arrangements are made for an on-site visit. The board of review then analyzes all of the information, and a letter with questions, comments, or recommendations is mailed to the agency.[7]

### Accounting

It is suggested that the accrual method be used for the accounting of home health agencies.[8] There are two major aspects involved in this type of accounting: the patient identification record and the visiting report.

The patient identification record should consist of patient's name, address, primary and secondary payment sources, patient number (preferably by I.D. plate), referral source, date of admission, diagnosis, census tract, and any other pertinent demographic information. It is important to know if the patient is new or a readmission. Distinct from patient treatment information, the patient information record is the basis for all financial and statistical information.

The visiting report, which is completed by the health professional, contains basic statistical and medical information. It should be completed immediately after the visit and should include mileage for employee reimbursement.

## Receiving Federal Money for Home Health Services

For twelve years, recipients covered under the Medicare program have been eligible for home health care reimbursement by the federal government. The following assumptions have been substantiated:

• Home health care is for the most part less expensive than institutional care.
• The population would prefer care provided within the home.
• There is a significant need/demand for home health care beyond the capacity of resources nationwide.[9]

Recognizing that the nation could not adequately provide home health services to population groups that were entitled to these benefits under existing legislation (i.e., Medicare and Medicaid), Congress authorized the Home Health Service Program under Public Law 94–63, Section 602. The secretary of Health, Education, and Welfare is authorized to make grants for the following purposes:

• meeting the initial cost of establishing home health agencies
• expanding the services available through existing home health agencies
• compensating personnel during the period of initial operation or agency expansion[10]

If a home health agency is to receive P.L. 94–63 monies, the agency must meet Medicare requirements for certification (NLN-APHA standards). If an agency is awarded a grant and does not meet the Medicare requirements for certification, that agency is given sixty days to comply with the requirements of certification. Furthermore, grants are awarded for a period of up to seventeen months, if necessary, to provide sufficient time for the applicant to achieve an operational level that will support the continued provision of home health services in the area.

P.L. 94–63 requires that preference in the awarding of grants be given areas within a state in which a sizable proportion of the population to be served is elderly, medically indigent, or both. Preference areas are as follows:

• percentage of individuals aged sixty-five years or over
• percentage of individuals with annual income below the poverty level
• percentage of individuals aged sixty-five years and older who live in poverty[11]

Federal responsibility for the Home Health Service Program belongs to the Bureau of Community Health Services of the Health Service Administration. During fiscal years 1976 and 1977, the department funded 112 projects with a total of $6 million. "Approximately 85 percent of the appropriated monies went to grant awards for the development or expansion of Home Health Agencies in preference areas."[12]

The establishing of a home health agency involves a process designed to maintain quality and consistency nationwide in the provision of home health care services. This is an ongoing process, and the conditions and regulations governing home health agencies may be expected to change as time goes on. For those desiring the most up-to-date information concerning home health care, and more specifically the accreditation of home health agencies, the National League of Nursing would be the best place to start.

# 7

# HOW TO FACILITATE
# HOME HEALTH CARE

The first step in the facilitation of home health care involves choosing the requirements necessary for a client's recovery, This depends on the seriousness of the client's illness. But whatever the case, a client participating in a home health care program will need what is referred to as a home health care triad (HHC triad). The HHC triad consists mainly of the client's family, a nurse, and a physician.

For many reasons, which will be explained later, it is very important for the client's family to participate in caring for their loved one. This can be achieved through the instruction and guidance the nurse provides. But participation does not have to end with the family; anybody, from friends and relatives to neighbors, can also contribute.[2]

The second part of the HHC triad is the HHC nurse. As mentioned previously, the nurse instructs the family, friends, and anybody else involved in proper HHC techniques to insure quality care to the client.[3] Most important, the nurse is the professional who provides and supervises medication to the client (as prescribed by a physician).

The physician completes the HHC triad by prescribing and providing medical services to the client. Another vital responsibility of the physician is to approve and manage a client's HHC program in its entirety.[4]

## The Family

The first part of the HHC triad consists of the client's family. The family plays an important role in the client's recovery and treatment by providing the most comfort. One of the reasons HHC exists is so the client can recover and receive treatment in familiar surroundings — the home.[5] By avoiding the impersonal atmosphere of institutionalization, the client can remain in his or her own "natural habitat." HHC encourages recovery as quickly as possible, and with a strong chance for success.

The family can participate in a HHC program in more ways than one. First, because the family is knowledgeable on a client's personal needs, the chances of depression and demoralization can be minimized. The family can encourage the client and raise morale. Second, the family can also learn how to provide client care from another member of the HHC triad, the nurse.[6] The nurse can teach the family many procedures, such as changing the bedridden client's position for comfort, relieving client tension by massage, and making sure that client is given the prescribed medication on time.

By being involved, not only is the family assisting the nurse (leaving time for other important matters), but also gaining a sense of belonging. By contributing to a loved one — the client — the family's feelings of frustration and helplessness can be minimized. Participation allows the family to feel more in control of the client's situation and secure. Should any emergency arise, the family is able to handle it properly.

Participation in an HHC program can benefit the family even *after* treatment has terminated. By possessing the experience, knowledge, and skill learned from participating, the family can encourage relatives, friends, and neighbors when a loved one is ill, thus easing any feelings of confusion and sadness that they may have.

## Nursing

The nurse, the second part of the HHC triad, is perhaps the most important aspect of client care. The nurse is the specialist most likely to spend a great deal of time with the client. One of the nurse's many responsibilities when involved in an HHC program is to assist the client in regaining utmost personal health. The nurse must also possess good technical nursing skills. Client assessment is a skill that is vital to the improvement of the client's health. The nurse must be aware of what state the client's mental and emotional health is in.[7]

The client's mental health is an important factor in his or her chances for recovery. The client should possess a positive attitude throughout treatment, which will in turn further cooperation with the HHC triad.

The client must also maintain a sense of dignity at *all* times. This will help the client feel hope and appreciation rather than helplessness or loneliness.

Also important to the HHC nurse is a combination of technical skills, knowledge, and experience. With these skills the nurse should be able to determine what a client needs at any time. This is vital because the home health care nurse does not have the backup that hospital nurses have.[8] The HHC nurse is isolated; there are not other consultants — physicians or nurses — to give advice immediately.

While caring for a client, the nurse must be able to respond calmly and positively to any situation. Not only is the danger of physical damage reduced, but also of *death*. For example, instead of panicking, a nurse must be able to help a client who is suffering from a seizure. With experience, the HHC nurse should be able to act efficiently and effectively in any situation, no matter how acute.

The ability to teach others is another requirement of the HHC nurse. The nurse must be able to teach the client's family, friends, neighbors, and anybody else involved in the client's care such methods as how to lift and move a patient (to prevent bed sores), how to position a client't pillow (to enhance comfort), and the best times and weather in which to take a client outside (to break monotony).[9]

Teaching the family is important to an HHC program, not only because it completes the HHC triad, but because it minimizes any helplessness the family may feel about not being able to aid their ill loved one. The family helps the nurse by performing basic duties, which allows the nurse to expend energy on other more technical tasks. Most of all, teaching the family skills can minimize the danger in an acute situation, if one should arise during the nurse's absence.

Client evaluation is also essential. The nurse must be able to analyze a client's progress throughout treatment, and then inform the physician of the improvement or decline of the client's health.[10] From such reports, the physician decides if and what should be changed in a program, according to the client's needs.

Effective program coordination is another responsibility of the HHC nurse. Being able to deal and work in harmony with the client, as well as with the other individuals involved, facilitates the program. The nurse also must be aware of people's emotional needs and such basics as privacy.[11]

Two techniques of nursing exist. With the first, direct care, every duty from instruction to medical care, is performed by the nurse who provides personal care to the client. The second, indirect care, involves a nurse who provides care only periodically or whenever needed. The nurse also provides advice and instruction to those involved in care. One warning: even though the family can be taught many duties, it is useless and dangerous for the nurse to teach and expect the family to perform duties that require professional attention, such as injections, changing of catheters, or dressing changes (burn clients, especially, are very susceptible to infection). The most common method of care for a client under indirect care is to monitor and evaluate the client's records for progress. By doing this, the consultant nurse is able to advise and recommend what is needed to the physician.[12]

In HHC there are two different types of nurses. The first, the clinical nurse specialist (CNS), is educated and trained at the masters level. The CNS possesses a high level of knowledge in particular areas, such as certain age groups, psychology, rehabilitation, hospice care, body systems and organs. Special knowledge can prove to be very valuable.[13] For example, one nurse may specialize in treating infants, and another in the elderly. There is an obvious difference in the need of the two groups.

As another example, a client with an emotional problem such as being unable to cope with the aftereffects of breast surgery, can benefit greatly from a nurse with specialization in psychology. The nurse is trained to deal with the challenge of raising the client's morale. Another type of nurse, on the other hand, might be unable to cope with this client's problem and might exhibit frustration toward the client, thus lessening the quality of care given.

Specialization in hospice care is also very valuable. The nurse would be qualified to discuss this kind of program with the client, rather than merely avoid it as another nurse might. Such avoidance only encourages other caretakers to do the same. It is the client who suffers — and the quality of home health care. The ultimate defeat is with the purpose of home health care — to make clients as comfortable as possible in their "natural habitat."[14]

A specialization in the body systems and organs is useful, for example, to a client recovering at home from a heart-related operation. In case of an emergency, the nurse would know how to respond, possibly saving a life.

The second type of HHC nurse, the nurse practitioner, is not as highly trained and specialized as a clinical nurse specialist. The nurse practitioner is nonetheless an asset to HHC for such skills as being able to judge a client's state of health.[15] For example, if the client is suffering from a stroke, the nurse practitioner may not be able to treat the client, but could immediately advise the physician of the problem and possibly minimize the extent of damage.

The nurse practitioner is also able to carry out tasks family members are unable to fulfill, tasks so routine that a physician need not be present. This enables the physician to tend to other responsibilities.

The nurse practitioner's job is directed more toward personal care and less toward teaching. Most nurse practitioners possess the skills to handle the psychological needs of clients, such as emotional support and rehabilitation,[16] but because of lack of knowledge they are not as useful as clinical nurse specialists.

## Homemaker–Home Health Aide

Another service that helps facilitate home health care is the homemaker–home health aide. The HHC aide is trained to perform such duties as personal hygiene of the client and housekeeping. Personal hygiene includes brushing a client's hair, shaving male clients, and brushing teeth. Housekeeping duties include laundry, housecleaning, and preparation of meals.[17]

Personal hygiene is vital for the morale and maintenance of a client's dignity. By maintaining the client's appearance, the possibility of depression and loss of identity is minimized. And by maintaining an organized household, the client is able to reside in comfortable and unchanged surroundings, familiar before illness.

## The Physician

The physician completes the HHC triad. The physician plays a vital role as leader, adviser, and consultant to the client's overall HHC plan. The physician has final approval of any proposed HHC treatment plan. Before approval, the physician must make sure that the plan is appropriate to the client's needs; if not, the physician changes and recommends any other treatment or medication beneficial to the client.[18]

Once the HHC plan is approved and implemented, the physician must be informed of the client's progress. This is important for success-ful recovery because the physician adapts the treatment according to the progress or changes in the client's health status. For example, the physician would decrease a client's medication when recovery is nearly complete. Physician involvement in home health care depends on the client's needs. If a client is recovering from a life-threatening illness, the physician will most likely be actively involved.[19]

## Methods of Financing Home Health Care

A significant way of facilitating home health care would be to ac-quire financial assistance. Because of the inability to finance their care, many clients are unable to receive HHC. Another cause of dep-rivation is the lack of programs available for funding. The result has either been institutionalization of the client or a low-quality of HHC,[20] which defeats its purpose. Both of these alternatives lead to negative results in the client's welfare. However, many methods have been devised to finance costs, thus enabling the client to participate in HHC.

The first alternative discussed earlier, is Medicare which went into effect July 1, 1966. Consisting of two parts, the first, Part A, was de-vised to provide basic coverage of hospital and related posthospital care costs for the elderly and disabled. This part, entitled "Hospital Insurance Benefits for the Aged and Disabled," also covers HHC. Those partly covered are short-term, skilled services (physicians, nurses, etc.) costs for the client recovering from acute injury or illness. To qualifiy under this part, the client must have stayed in the hospital at least three days.[21]

The disadvantage of Medicare is that it only covers short-term HHC. This is useless, given that HHC mainly benefits those clients who need long recuperation periods, which are obviously more of a financial burden than short-term periods. Besides, short-term re-covery is usually accomplished in an institution.

Part B helps solve this problem. Supplementary to Part A, it is more advantageous in that it provides full coverage for such HHC costs as physician, nurse, and homemaker–home health aide. It also differs from Part A in that it must be purchased on a monthly basis.[22] The client is thus free to buy any amount of care desired.

To qualify for Medicare, however, there are criteria that a client must meet. Those eligible for benefits usually fall into one of two categories: clients over sixty-five years who are eligible for Social Security benefits, and disabled clients under the age of sixty-five who have been disabled for more than twenty-four months. Once eligible, recipients are entitled to coverage of services such as nursing, physical therapy, speech therapy, occupational therapy, medical supplies and appliances, and social service.[23]

The specific requirements of Part A are that a client must be home-bound, hospitalized at least three days, and treatment needed at home is for the same illness as that which caused institutionalization. The requirements of Part B are the same, with the exception of the mandatory three-day hospitalization period.[24]

A second way an HHC client can receive financial assistance is through Medicaid. Under Title XIX of the Social Security Act, Medicaid was enacted at about the same time as Medicare.[25] Funds exist under this program that are specifically allocated for home health care.

Under Medicaid, the federal government requires that each state devise its own HHC plan and administer it; thus plans differ from state to state. The services an eligible person receives are the same as with Medicare. Medicaid differs in the respect that eligibility cannot be based on whether a client was institutionalized before HHC was recommended. This is advantageous because it minimizes the cost of HHC from the start, by not requiring institutionalization in order to qualify. The disadvantage is that in many states the cost of care far exceeds reimbursement amount. This presents potential financial burdens for the HHC client.[26]

Another method of financing HHC is through private insurance. HHC benefits are part of most private health insurance policies. Most of the benefits provided in federally subsidized plans are available through private insurance, for instance, for such services as nursing, physical therapy, speech pathology, homemaker–home health aides, and medical supplies. There is usually a limit on the amount of visits over a period of time, when the program is indirect, for example, thirty visits over a period of forty-five days. Insurance policies may also extend or decrease this limitation, depending on the seriousness of a patient's illness.[27]

The Veterans Administration is another financial provider for those clients who have served in the armed forces. Services available include physician care, nursing, homemaker–home health aide, rehabilitation, and social worker care. A veteran benefits greatly from the services offered because the Veterans Administration holds the philosophy that the client will recuperate more quickly if placed in a familiar environment—the home.[28]

## Services Facilitating Home Health Care

Meals delivered at home, transportation, and friendly visitors are nonprofessional services to help support and maintain an HHC client's morale. The client without a family is the one who benefits the most from this type of service. Home health care would be useless if the client did not have positive feelings and was preoccupied by something other than the goal of successful recovery.

Meals delivered at home (e.g., "Meals-on-Wheels") provide the client with a well-balanced, nutritious, and one hopes good-tasting meal.[29] Clients receiving this service are usually unable to prepare their own meals or have no one else to do it for them. With Meals-on-Wheels not only is the client able to receive three meals a day, but also a chance to talk to somebody other than the primary caregiver.

Meals-on-Wheels are usually sponsored by a client's community, church, or a private organization specializing in meal preparation.[30]

Transportation is another service that facilitates HHC by providing mobility to the client. Because clients are often in an HHC setting to save money, they usually cannot afford transportation. Whether the transportation be taxi, bus, or private chauffeur service, the problem still exists: cost. Providing transportation ensures that the client will receive whatever treatment must be done in a hospital, for example, a series of tests.[32]

A Friendly Visitor service is another voluntary program that helps the client.[33] This service would apply specifically to the client without a family. Without somebody to talk to, a client's morale can easily deteriorate, causing serious depression, which in turn may prolong a client's recovery. As previously explained, a positive attitude is necessary for a client's recovery to go as smoothly as possible. With this service, a client has somebody to talk to and play cards with, even to go shopping with if not bedridden. The client without a family benefits immensely from the Friendly Visitor service.

## Conclusion

As we have seen, a variety of services are available that make home health care possible for many seeking an alternative to institutionalization. Many costs incurred can be paid, at least in part, by federal programs such as Medicare and Medicaid. Other financial assistance services include private insurance and, for those who have served in the armed forces, the Veterans Administration.

It is the HHC triad of family, nurse, and physician that eases a client's recovery. The family facilitates the program by providing comfort to the client and encouragement for a quick recovery, as well as carrying out certain treatment duties. This helps the nurse and doctor, and the family too, by allowing them to contribute to their loved one's care.

The nurse, whether *"direct"* or *"indirect"* is always teaching those involved in the program methods that will maximize comfort and quality care of the client.

The physician provides medical care to the client. The extent to which the physician is involved depends on the case. Involvement is greater, for instance, if a patient is recovering from a serious illness or operation. Approval of a client's HHC program rests with the physician.

# 8

# HOME BIRTH: AN OLD PRACTICE IN REJUVENATION

T he hospital is the workplace of physicians; it contains all the tools of their trade and the facilities with which to apply their craft. The hospital is also the refuge of the ill. A great majority of Americans do not think about their health until it's lost — and then they have to go to the hospital so a physician can find it and "give it back." Pregnancy and birth are glorious experiences of life that, although beautiful, can present dangers to both the mother and child. In the last century, the place of birth has changed drastically from the home to the hospital. Whenever illness strikes or health dangers arise, the hospital is assumed to be the place to be because of professional facilities, equipment, and staff. Recently, there has been a growing interest in the issue of the birth setting, which includes four elements: the locale, the recipients of care, the providers of maternity care, and the practice of those providers.

In 1900, only 5 percent of all babies were delivered in hospitals. A little over forty years ago, half of all births occurred at home and half in hospitals. But today, 99 percent of all babies are born in hospitals. Providers of maternity care have changed also. In 1910, lay midwives delivered 50 percent of all babies; by 1979, they only delivered 1.6 percent of all infants, whereas physicians delivered 98.1 percent of all hospital births as well as 34.2 percent of those born elsewhere.[1] Why are hospitals the dominant birth setting now? Is planned home birth a good alternative? Why the concern over the birth setting? These are some of the questions being raised on this issue.

As has been noted, the place of birth has changed drastically in just the last forty years. This change alone is enough to spark interest in health care delivery analysts, but the real catalysts of the birth setting review come from the women's movement, consumerism, the desire for a natural delivery, and concern over rising costs. This has created two predominant schools of thought: advocates and opponents of alternative birth settings. Advocates have succeeded in turning some of their ideas into reality in the form of independent birth centers, in-hospital birth centers, clinics, and home delivery services. This chapter will examine the home as an alternative place of birth. It is appropriate to begin by analyzing past developments that affect us today.

## History

Between 1910 and 1912, Abraham Flexner and J. W. Williams cited obstetrics as the weakest specialty.[2] This revelation raised concern within the profession and action was taken to improve service in this field. Obstetricians centered their efforts on four areas: the high rate of maternal mortality, relief of pain during childbirth, high neonatal mortality, and, more recently, the psychological well-being of the mother, as well as of the infant.

The main cause of the drastic increase in the proportion of births occurring in hospitals was improvements in obstetrical practice. Obstetricians knew the public health problems, what needed to be done, and how to go about doing it. They improved their services and accomplished what they set out to do in the areas of maternal and neonatal mortality. Between 1955 and 1980, maternal mortality decreased from 47 to 7 deaths per 100,000 live births. Neonatal deaths during this same period decreased from 19.1 to 8.4 per 100,000 births.[3]

Needless to say, the statistics reflect improved safety and quality of care during childbirth. Obviously, parents want the safest delivery possible, hence the attraction to hospitals and professional assistance, often referred to as the "medicalization" of childbirth. It represents a gradual shift in viewpoint, with pregnancy increasingly being considered an illness.

A complementary trend is increased use of obstetrical procedures. The use of induced labor increased from 8.6 percent to 11.8 percent of all births during the ten-year period between 1967 and 1977. Similarly, cesarean sections increased from 7.3 percent to 13.4 percent of births during the five-year span between 1972 and 1977.[5] Obstetricians also integrated anesthesia and analgesia during childbirth to reduce pain and thus alleviate much of the fear of childbirth. It is difficult to say whether or not this trend is beneficial, nevertheless, it is the contention of alternative birth setting advocates that women should be able to avoid such unnatural interferences with the birth process if they so choose.

## Birth at Home as an Alternative to the Hospital

Because of our dependency on hospitals, the home is now considered only an "option" for some parents, although for a few people it is the unplanned delivery locale when, for one reason or another, they can't get to the hospital in time. Planned home birth is the aspect of nonconventional maternity care that generates the most concern among professionals and the most controversy between providers and consumers.

The first question that comes to mind is, "Why birth at home?" In a study made of two groups of women in Salt Lake County, Utah, who planned their deliveries to be at home, the women were asked why they wanted to give birth in their homes. The five most prevalent answers were:

- control of their delivery
- to have a family-centered experience
- to eliminate interferences with normal processes
- personalized care
- low cost

Autonomy and psychological ideals are the main reasons for home birth. It has been charged that home birth is an alternative geared mainly to the underprivileged because of their financial constraints. This simply is not so. A great majority of parents who plan births at home do so mainly out of a desire to control the delivery and treat it as a family experience.[6]

A fundamental element in determining whether the home is a safe alternative is risk assessment. Women who wish to give birth at home should be screened for indications of possible conditions that may preclude home birth because they cause unnecessary risks to both mother and child. If the woman is advised, through risk assessment, not to give birth at home, she should search for other available birth settings that meet her needs.

In a study made of home deliveries in North Carolina from 1974 to 1976, the investigators determined whether the deliveries were planned or unplanned, whether there was a trained birth attendant (a lay midwife), and whether prenatal care and screening were performed. They found that the women attended by lay midwives had been classified by prenatal screening as medically low-risk pregnancies. Planned home deliveries not attended by lay midwives had not been similarly screened.

Prenatally screened women, in spite of their high-risk demographic profile (e.g., poor, little education), had the lowest neonatal mortality (3 per 1,000 births). But women who were not prenatally screened had a higher neonatal mortality rate (30 per 1,000 live births), in spite of their low-risk demographic profile (e.g., not poor, more education). The neonatal mortality rate among unplanned home delivery was the highest (120 per 1,000 live births).[7]

Risk-assessment instruments must clearly differentiate between high- and low-risk groups with a sensitivity of no less than 80 percent.[8] Sensitivity is an indication of the screening method's ability to identify correctly those women with a given disease or condition. Specificity is an indication of the screening method's ability to identify correctly those women without a given condition.

It is estimated that between 36,000 and 158,000 babies were delivered outside hospitals in 1980. Births at home comprised 1 percent of all births.[9] It is a small proportion, and the literature does not suggest that the percentage of home births will increase in the very near future. Medicalization is a social phenomenon that is difficult to avoid once established.

Lay midwives deliver about half of all babies born at home, and physicians deliver a bit more than a third. The remainder of home deliveries are unattended. In some parts of the country home delivery services are offered to the public. These services range from a solitary lay midwife to a delivery team including an attending physician. However, considering that only 1 percent of all babies are born out of hospitals, these services are having little impact on birthing practices. Of course, that's not to say that they won't in the future.

## Is Home Birth Safe?

To answer the question of safety, a physician or screening instrument must identify any health factors that indicate home birth is an unwise option. If, by professional judgment, there is no apparent risk to giving birth at home (although there is, of course, always a degree of risk), then it might be a worthy alternative. Naturally, appropriate provisions must be made for possible complications.

In a very detailed study of the medical records of 1,146 home births attended by five northern California home delivery services between 1970 and 1975, which included data on demography, attendants, population served, process of care, outcome, and complications, the study team compared the incidence of various events recorded at the home births to the birth population of the state as reported in the literature. The home births sustained zero maternal deaths and the prenatal mortality rate of 9.5 per 1,000 was lower than the state average.[10] Critics charge that the study group was self-selected. In fact, the lower mortality rate illustrates that the group was, indeed, self-selected through a process of careful screening, which clearly indicated the safety or low risk of birth at home. The screening method used was sensitive and specific.

In another carefully planned study, close attention was paid to variables known to be associated with pregnancy outcome. Medical records of 1,046 home births in northern California and Madison, Wisconsin, were compared to an equal number of births from two community hospitals in Madison. Both groups were pair-matched for maternal age, education, parity, gestation age, major risk factors, and total risk score. Both populations were upper middle class and 98 percent white.

Although posterior delivery and bleeding during labor occurred more often in home births, the research team found no significant difference in neonatal and fetal mortality, number of neurologically abnormal infants, and the incidence of low birth weight. However, women who gave birth in hospitals received significantly more intravenous oxytocin, anethesia, and analgesia; more low- and mid-forcep deliveries, cesareans, episotomies, and lacerations. These women also had more labor and delivery complications, elevated blood pressure, dystocia, and postpartum hemorrhaging. The infants sustained more birth injuries, fetal distress, meconium staining, total oxygen administered, and respiratory distress syndrome inside hospitals.[11]

These data suggest that not only are home births safe, but clinical iatrogenesis may be an obscure incentive to avoid the hospital and give birth at home if possible. If a woman has decided to relinquish the benefits of the hospital in favor of the home, she also trades the risks of hospital birth to those of the home method. Mehl and Peterson could not find evidence to support the hypothesis that the risks of home birth outweigh those of the conventional method.

## Psychological Considerations of Childbirth

In the past, women gave birth to their children at home. There, among family and friends, they were not "patients" and childbirth was not an illness. It was a natural process — but too often unsafe.[14] Although modern birth methods offer safety, the atmosphere is often associated with illness and suffering and lacks the warmth and reassurance that the home provides. A frequent complaint of the conventional birth is that often the woman is not given an opportunity to establish a personal bond with her infant immediately after birth, and families are not treated as a cohesive unit or given any role in decision making.[12]

Advocates of home birth believe that their method offers significant psychological advantages to the parents, the newborn infant, and its siblings. They especially believe that the bonding between baby and mother can take place more easily at home in a relaxed environment, surrounded by familiar and supportive attendants.[13] Some favor home birth because of unpleasant experiences with earlier births in a hospital. Many of them had little choice in their birthing method or their activities during labor; they could not have any family present or have sufficient access to their baby following birth. They believed the hospital and their physicians were authoritarian and impersonal. Many are concerned that there may be excessive intervention in what they consider to be a natural event. Some believe that childbirth is not inherently dangerous and should not take place in hospitals that are oriented to the care of the ill.[14]

It is evident that planning the birth setting requires thoughtful consideration of one's priorities well in advance of the event.

## Role of the Midwife

Midwifery is possibly the world's oldest profession; it goes back one million years. The midwife's services, however, have declined sharply in the last eighty years due to increased physician involvement in the birth process, the medicalization of childbirth, and more. But another very significant setback for midwives was the enactment of state laws prohibiting midwives from using the tools of the medical trade.

Nevertheless, the primary tools of midwives and the key to successful home births are patience and preparation. The midwife allows the birth to proceed at its natural pace and refuses to rush the process. "If the birth takes fifteen or forty minutes, that's okay," says midwife Norman Casserley. Unlike the midwife, the physician must follow a schedule and certain standards set by the American College of Obstetricians and Gynecologists. Each stage of the birth should take a specific amount of time, and if these standards are not met, the doctor may employ artificial measures to stick to the norm.[15]

If a decision is made to give birth at home, it would probably be easier to find a qualified midwife rather than a willing physician or obstetrician.

## Summary and Conclusions

The concern over the birth setting is twofold: parents are concerned that not all of their needs are satisfied by the conventional birth method, and the professional medical care provider community is concerned that home birth is unsafe, although there is no evidence to support this claim. Professionals do have control of the childbirth market, which must indicate that alternative birth setting advocates must take a stand, conduct studies or have them contracted to be done, educate the public, and publicize their service if they want to have an impact on childbirth practices and attitudes.

Allowing for thorough screening and preparation, home birth does appear to be a safe alternative to the hospital. Both the hospital and the home have their unique benefits and risks; however, there is little, if any, objective evidence on the advantages or disadvantages of any birth setting.[17] Parents must use careful consideration in making a birth-setting decision. Those who opt for home birth are advised to seek professional guidance in the form of home delivery services or a midwife and spend ample time and effort in preparation.

Because of their concern for safety, professionals are unlikely to put themselves in what they view as a precarious position. The lay midwife has been and still is the key to home birth. The midwife is the instructor of birth methods, the confidant, the attendant, and the source of trust, friendship, and guidance.

Home delivery is an alternative that presents benefits and risks, the greater of which must be considered by the individual parents. It has been estimated, however, that if home delivery service providers delivered a quarter of all babies born annually, the service would be viable, as good as the present system, with total reduction in cost to the general consumer public.[18]

# 9

# THE FUTURE OF HOME BIRTH
# IN THE UNITED STATES

There is a growing movement toward greater awareness in dealing with modern medicine. It has been only recently (the past twenty years or so) that the average citizen has thought of questioning the "supreme" knowledge of the physician. Physicians have traditionally enjoyed such high regard by society that their motives and practices were never questioned. This is changing, however. The patient of the 1980s wants to know all the relevant issues and reasons regarding the medical treatment he or she receives. People are tired of complying passively with technical assaults on their bodies in the name of medical science. Their dissatisfaction has forced physicians to acknowledge their right as patients to be informed. Physicians aren't necessarily enthusiastic about these changes, but they are bit by bit realizing that people want to be active partners in decision making regarding their consumption of medical services. This has resulted in a wider variety of health care alternatives for consumers.

This chapter will focus on an alternative to the institution, i.e., home care. Home care can be defined as the delivery of medical services to a patient in the home. This definition is extremely broad. To narrow it a bit, home care often involves a different philosophy of the delivery of medical services, that is, a reduction of services. Home care has come to symbolize the use of medical services and personnel at the absolute minimum level of intervention. This type of care is characterized by greater sensitivity on the part of the health service personnel. Medical services provided in the home are ideally only those that are absolutely necessary to the patient's health or comfort. There have been numerous studies comparing health service treatments delivered in the hospital and in the home setting. These studies raise certain questions: is the quality of care provided in the home equivalent to, better than, or worse than that provided in the hospital? This chapter will address these and other such questions concerning childbirth. The different services currently available will be examined so as to observe any qualitative differences between them.

## Recent Trends in Child Delivery

At present about 1 to 3 percent of all deliveries occur at home.[1] Although the majority of deliveries are in the hospital, there is a growing acceptance of home childbirth. Why the recent upsurge in home delivery? Most likely it is due to better education of today's patients and their concern over the increased use of technology in obstetrics. Probably one of the greatest reasons for concern is the rising incidence of cesarean section delivery. A cesarean section (known as a C-section) is a surgical procedure performed by the obstetrician to deliver a child in the event of dangerous complications. A C-section is supposed to be a last resort used to save the life of the child or the mother. The decision on whether or not a situation is life threatening rests solely with the physician. Not only does technology play a large role in physicians' interpretation of what constitutes danger, but recently the motives upon which these decisions are based have been questioned.

Over the past twenty years, the number of C-sections has risen substantially. In fact, during this period the percentage of C-sections performed has tripled.[2] This is an alarming figure, considering the implications this has on mother and child, both physically and emotionally. In a study published in the October 1980 issue of the *British Journal of Obstetrics*, it was revealed that during a three-month audit of obstetric practices in a British hospital, the incidence of C-sections decreased significantly. This implies that there is considerable discretion on the part of the physician in choosing such a procedure.

Dr. Robert Mendelsohn, in his book *Confessions of a Medical Heretic*, states that *most* C-sections are physician induced. Dr. Mendelsohn asserts that *most* obstetricians manipulate their patients' deliveries so as to fit them into proper physicians' office hours. This view is also supported by R. Goodlin in a study in which he found that "C-sections occurred at certain times of the day and hardly at other times." This may seem like earth-shaking news to the public, but it is not to obstetricians. "They inform us that everyone knows that elective induction of labor is a common practice. They wonder why we choose to point it out. When we discuss our findings with nonmedical persons, we get a very different reaction. They cannot imagine the practice is as common as we show it is." This is frightening news to most women contemplating a hospital delivery. Modern medicine treats pregnancy as an illness, since that is what institutions were built to handle. To simply guide a woman through a biologically normal process like childbirth is too passive a role for medical personnel.

Goodlin's study supports the view that the presence of sophisticated technology in the hospital poses a threat, not a help, to the majority of mothers who need no medical intervention. The reason is clear: elective induction of labor poses a substantial risk to both mother and child. "A labor induced by the doctor can end up a cesarean section delivery, because the baby that is not ready to be born will naturally show more distress on fetal monitors, distress at being summoned prematurely." There is no end to the number of studies on the impact of electronic fetal monitors and their results on the percentage of C-sections performed. Obstetricians are increasing their use of fetal monitoring for a number of reasons: the desire to base their actions on objective clinical data, the "scientific" value of more information, and the medical/legal concern with not using a technique that many obstetricians say is necessary. Whatever the reason, one thing is clear: electronic fetal monitoring is not beneficial to the great majority of obstetrical patients.[3]

Two studies on electronic fetal monitors (EFM) over a four-year period showed that their use resulted in no significant drop in fetal morbidity or mortality. It was enlightening to note, however, that in both studies the group using EFM equipment had three times the number of cesarean deliveries as the control group.[4] Fetal monitoring may give the physician more information, but more information does not necessarily produce better results. For example, the data from this study suggest that some women are undergoing unnecessary cesarean sections, while at the same time the costs of delivery are going from $700 to $3,000.

Many obstetricians simply can't resist the temptation to turn an ordinary delivery into a major surgical procedure, with the increased fees that go along with it. Perhaps this is why they favor electronic fetal monitors so much. If the mother doesn't want a cesarean, all the physician has to do is point to the distressed blips on the monitor screen. It forces patient compliance. Dr. Mendelsohn has proposed we change the name from fetal monitoring to *fatal* monitoring. After all, EFM's don't really ensure any greater level of safety for the baby; they just triple the chance of cesarean delivery.

An interesting point on cesarean section: although obstetricians claim a reduced perinatal mortality rate as a result of increased cesarean section: studies have proven otherwise. Also it has been noted that in other countries there has been a decline in fetal deaths without any increase in C-sections.[5]

There are other negative trends in child delivery that have been forced on women: chemical stimulation of labor, drugs administered before and after birth, use of X-rays and ultrasound, separation of mother from familial support during labor. It is not known which of these procedures might be imposed on a patient unnecessarily, but the prospect is enough to make many prospective mothers look for an alternative. The alternative many are considering is home childbirth.

## Home Birth as an Alternative

Considering some of the procedures just discussed, it is no wonder that some women question whether hospitals are in the best interest of mothers and families giving birth. Birth is a very personal thing. There should be safe, sensible choices in determining the way women want to deliver. "If we are to produce a normal generation of children with normal intelligence, we must begin now to find safe alternatives in childbirth for low risk mothers and their babies in order that they will not become high risk as a result of their care in the hospital."[6] Home birth is one answer to the need for alternatives. It involves the philosophy of viewing birth as a natural process that shouldn't be disturbed by any unnecessary medical practices. To outline this concept, home birth is characterized by: comfortable homelike surroundings; presence of the husband and other family members; natural birth procedure, which avoids any interventionist obstetric practices; promotion of emotional bonding between child and mother through lack of separation after birth, attendance by midwife.

Home childbirth can take place in the woman's home, in a simulated home setting in the hospital, or in a "freestanding" birthing center not connected to a hospital. In 1973, there were three such facilities (small, comfortable birthing centers with some emergency equipment). Now there are 130 of them in 27 states. In most home births the delivery is performed by a nurse or a midwife. This is not to say that physicians never do them. For the most part, however, this type of delivery is not favored by the medical community. (We will discuss some of the reasons for this in a later section.)

In the 1700s, the vast majority of deliveries were performed by midwives, a woman trained in assisting the natural course of childbirth. These women did not hold any type of medical degree, and this is probably the reason they began to be pushed out of practice by men in the late 1700s. Male practitioners were then introduced, on the premise that they were well educated and knowledgeable on anatomy. It was thought that male practitioners would improve the child delivery process, but, in fact, "the introduction of men into the business of reproductive management brought special dangers to mothers and babies." Many women are simply more comfortable having their babies delivered with the help of another woman. Although there are legions of male obstetricians who feel they are experts in the field of childbirth, who should know more about the process than a woman who has experienced it? For this reason, home birth advocates point to the greater understanding and sensitivity the midwife has for the woman's condition. In Madera County, California, ten years ago, the state supported a project that introduced midwives into that community. After one year, the infant mortality rate was reduced from 23.9 per 1000 live births, to 10.3. Prematurity dropped from 11 percent of all births to 6.4 percent. These midwives obviously proved that there was a great need for health care in that particular community. The project was dropped at the recommendation of the Health Department and the obstetricians of the state. Within six months birthing problems returned to the unusually high rate that had existed before the program was adopted. This study uncovers another issue in the practice of home birth as a viable alternative — safety.[7]

Advocates of home births cite this and other studies to back up their claim of safety. Hospital births versus home births have been studied in Sweden, Denmark, Holland, England, and the United States, with no distinct differences in results. This would certainly seem to indicate that home birth methods are at least as safe as hospital delivery. As a matter of fact, most statistics give home birth a clear edge over hospital birth with respect to infant mortality. One study by Dr. Lewis E. Mehl, comparing a California home birth program to the total perinatal death rate in California, showed that the home birth program was effective in reducing infant mortality from 20.3 percent to 9.5 percent. A study in North Carolina showed that home birth (planned, with an attending midwife) resulted in a four per thousand infant death rate, as opposed to a twelve per thousand rate in the hospital. Of the infant deaths that occurred in this study under the home birth program, 3 of the 4 percent were associated with congenital anomalies and may not have been preventable. It is important to note the significance of a preplanned home birth program with attending midwife, since as a result of this study it was revealed that the relative risk of unplanned home deliveries was twenty times that of planned home deliveries. This is significant because opponents of home birth see it as a primitive, reckless practice. To advocates of home birth this view is considered biased and wrongminded, because the theory of home birth is a comprehensive plan that involves much more than simply having a baby at home. Therefore, the argument for home births is invalid unless the program is accompanied by an appropriate prenatal education and a qualified nurse-midwife.[8]

To examine some of the statistics a bit further, it was observed in a Michigan study that birth weights for homeborns increased significantly over those of hospital deliveries. Not only did average weights rise, but mortality for high birth weight babies was reduced. The most likely reason for this is that in home birth techniques, there is no induced labor. The mother isn't forced into labor too early, and the baby is given a chance to fully mature. This has proven to be extremely beneficial to both mother and child, since labor doesn't start until both are prepared for it. It also aids in deterring a problem called "the lancet," i.e., "in any large series of elective deliveries at term, there will inevitably be a proportion of cases in which an error in the dating of gestation results in a premature child who may die or suffer irreparable damage in the neonatal period." Elective induction involves many negative effects and risks, such as prematurity, fetal hypoxia, risk to fetal head and long-term child development.[9]

These studies indicate how truly dangerous the common practice of elective induction is to both mother and child. The absence of this practice alone should be enough to favor endorsement of home birth by mothers coast to coast.

It is important to note that all subjects who participate in a home birth study are thoroughly screened. According to most doctors, about two-thirds of the mothers who stand a substantial risk of serious complications during labor can be identified well in advance and advised to have the baby in the hospital. As a result, high-risk mothers are virtually eliminated from home birth programs. Thus hospital deliveries include a much larger percentage of complicated cases, and the statistics reflect this. Of course we still don't know how many cases involving complications were *caused* by the physicians, but it does represent a small bias nonetheless.

To conclude this discussion of the safety aspects of home birth: most studies show a statistically significant decrease in overall neonatal mortality as a result of the program. Of course, physicians have hundreds of studies that prove otherwise (or so they believe), but there is no statistical proof to support the belief that home childbirth is dangerous. If you ask physicians what their main objection to home childbirth is, they will invariably tell you that it simply isn't safe. By the same token, home birth advocates will reply by pointing out the many obstetric practices they feel are relatively unsafe. "Whether home births are good or bad, however, can never be answered purely by statistical method — not only because the statistics are inadequate but also because value judgments are so important in this matter." Focusing on safety is a vital element of determining the worth of a particular medical procedure. In this case, however, it obscures the real issue. Home birth has proven to be a safe and satisfying alternative for many. Physicians still argue against it for reasons of safety, but the real issue is that physicians are trying to force one type of care on consumers. They refuse to offer people desperately needed alternatives. "Any time there is a monopoly of power, there is small incentive to make changes to fit peoples' needs. But if alternatives are provided, people may choose and this would encourage positive improvement in all alternatives."[10] What are some of the motives that move physicians to battle so actively against offering alternatives to consumers?

## Physicians—The Implications of Their Motives and Attitudes in the Delivery of Medical Services

Beginning with their early days in medical school, physicians are taught to practice medicine in a specific way. They are socialized into a modern medical philosophy that convinces them to utilize their knowledge and skills. It doesn't matter that the knowledge they attain and the skills they use are often inappropriate. Physicians are taught to *do* something. It makes them very uncomfortable to be confronted with a medical situation in which no level of intervention will help. Take, for example, physicians' treatment of cancer patients. At the onset of cancer, physicians welcome the challenge to use the full battery of chemical, surgical, and technological treatments at their disposal. When those treatments don't work and it is clear the disease will "run its course," the physician-patient relationship deteriorates. There are plenty of ways that the patient requires care even at this stage of the illness, e.g., pain control and emotional support. In spite of this, most physicians grow increasingly scarce at this stage, since the failure of the patient to get well indicates a weakness in the treatment. It is almost as if the physician says, "If I can't work my magic on you, I'll find someone it will work on."

This parallels the view of most of today's obstetricians. They go to school to learn how to perform all sorts of diagnostic and surgical techniques, which are only required in about 3 percent of all deliveries. What are they supposed to do the other 97 percent of the time? The answer is frightening!

When there isn't enough demand for obstetrical services, then demand must be stimulated, even if artificially. Not all physicians are crooks, but they are trained to utilize their education. It was expensive to obtain, and they have every intention of profiting from their labor.

If there is not a large enough outlet for their training, they will consciously or unconsciously manipulate demand. The result is unnecessary risks for obstetrical patients. It is commonly known that the more obstetricians who occupy a given area, the larger percentage of obstetric surgery there is in that area. Is the additional medical care really needed, or is it created? The implication is clear: physicians are educated for the purpose of practicing. The principles of modern medicine simply don't allow them to be simple observers. The following is a list of common obstetric practices for which there is no scientific support:

1. separating the mother from her family during labor and birth
2. routine medication

3. shaving of the perineum
4. electronic monitoring of the fetus
5. use of ultrasound
6. use of X-rays
7. routine episiotomy (making an incision to prevent vaginal tearing during labor)
8. use of stirrups
9. artificial formula instead of mother's milk[11]

Although not a single one of these common procedures can be scientifically defended, physicians will argue in their defense. This brings up the issue of the statistical discrepancy evident in studies of most of these procedures.

It seems that with a little creative accounting, you can interpret statistics to mean anything you desire. Thus, physicians justify their practices with studies that do not represent conclusive scientific evidence.

Why do physicians defend such questionable practices so fervently? Because they are established, and they are profitable. Established medical practices die hard, because doctors' organizations are powerful groups to contend with. For example, the American Medical Association seeks to prescribe and protect those practices that it feels should be accepted. It exists to serve physicians and patients alike, but it is no secret that if forced to choose, it will favor the interests of physicians. One of the major interests the AMA protects is physicians' income. For instance, in many states midwives represented such a threat to physicians' income that the AMA exerted political force to make it unlawful to practice midwifery.

Another example involves a general practitioner who became disillusioned with hospital births when he wasn't allowed to dim the lights or practice other natural childbirth techniques while helping his wife deliver their ninth child in a hospital. Dr. Wootan began practicing home childbirth shortly after that. When he performed a Leboyer birth, he was suspended for practicing a "radical new obstetric procedure." He pointed out that the procedure was being performed in other hospitals in the area and was reinstated, but his troubles weren't over. At the instigation of local doctors, the Board of Health began investigating him as "an imminent danger to the health of the people of New York State." Wootan filed suit against the Department of

Health. A month after his suspension, the State Supreme Court ruled that the suspension was "so unreasonable as to be arbitrary." The state Board of Health appealed and he was automatically resuspended. Of his case Wootan commented, "It opened my eyes to the biases against anything but established medicine."

At this point Wootan is being aided by a group of supporters who have formed a "friends of Wootan society" to help him raise money for his defense. In the past few years, five other doctors in New York State who have practiced home births have had to face charges of incompetence. They have either given up home births or gone underground. Wootan says he cost local hospitals $250,000 in lost fees since he began practicing home births — one reason for the fierce opposition of his colleagues.

A study of some of the wealthiest areas of the country — e.g., Grosse Pointe, Michigan; Scarsdale, New York; and Phoenix, Arizona — has revealed the incidence of learning disability in children there to be as high as one in four. There is no genetic or family predisposing factor in 75 percent of these cases.

It is obvious that we need alternatives to our present hospital maternity care. Mothers and families need to organize so their voices will be heard and physicians will realize they must put an end to many of their practices. "A dichotomy exists in obstetrics today between the technological trend represented in its extreme and couples planning home delivery without medical support. We feel that reducing the antagonism between these divergent poles would enhance care for women choosing hospital as well as home deliveries."[12]

To sum up, physicians' motives and attitudes are instrumental in determining the type of care available to patients today. Physicians need to be more receptive to alternative approaches, however, so as to assure the high quality of medical care that patients deserve.

## Perceptions of Quality

The decision for most mothers on whether to deliver at home or in the hospital is based on the qualitative differences in the two types of care. If physicians were more sensitive to what women perceive as quality care, there would be no controversy in this area.

After organizing a series of conferences ("Dialogues with Women"), it became obvious that "women's representatives meant something quite different from what physicians understand when speaking of the quality of medical care." The physician's concept of quality care is related to whether he or she has adequate training, experience to understand specific problems, ability to perceive complications in the early stages, and skill to correct these problems with generally good long-term results. On the other hand, when women speak of quality medical care, they most frequently recommend modifications in the environment surrounding the medical care: more warmth and personal considerateness; more empathy; less callous disregard; more willingness of the physician to inform the patient of her alternatives, to consult her, and to allow her to make some choices.

The birthing process that has existed for the past forty years hasn't allowed the mother any choices. In fact, it has infringed on her rights and exploited her. Home birth techniques have been increasingly accepted, but change hasn't come fast enough. "Sometimes a young couple would arrive at the hospital only to find that months of careful preparation for some form of 'natural childbirth' had been in vain because the obstetric staff was reluctant to cooperate."[13] This problem has particularly angered women, because they seem to have no control over what is done to their bodies. The result of this anger is a movement toward legal action called "informed consent." Informed consent is a legal and ethical doctrine that protects an individual's right to determine what shall be done to her body. It is in the power of the patient to bring charges of battery against a physician if he so much as touches her without her consent. It is sad to think that the public has become so suspicious of physicians that such a policy is necessary. It does, however, legally relay the message to physicians that patients are to be treated as autonomous, responsible individuals.

This is, in fact, the key to the whole concept of quality medical care — to include the patient in the process and to be sensitive to her feelings and needs. Many of the medical procedures performed in obstetrics have been to benefit the physician, not the patient. This is why women seek a higher quality alternative.

Is home childbirth the answer to the higher standards women are seeking? Studies and individual testimonies of women in home birth programs indicate that they are much more satisfied than those whose babies were delivered in hospitals. Maybe this is because the home birth program is tailored to the needs of the mother and family, not the medical staff. At home, there isn't the slightest possibility that the mother will have to undergo any unnecessary surgical intervention. And since tests have shown that mothers who delivered by cesarean section were "more likely to have difficulty establishing a relationship with their child," this can only be a benefit.[14]

There is, however, one problem with home birth that has not been solved. In those rare situations when mothers require emergency measures (about 3 percent of all births), it may be impossible to get to a hospital. This problem can be solved with home birth rooms within the hospital. More and more of them are being set up, much to the benefit of mothers. With these rooms, patients can have all the advantages of home birth—Leboyer methods, family participation, midwife delivery, lack of drugs or monitors—while maintaining the safety in emergency situations that the hospital can provide.

## The Future

It might be interesting to note that as I researched the medical journals for views on home births, I noticed a trend in physician-author attitudes. The articles from the early 1970s seemed to be more critical of the home birth movement. As the movement gained more and more support, there were a great number of articles criticizing physicians and their obstetric practices. The literature of the 1980s exhibits a widespread knowledge of the shortcomings of modern obstetric practices. Then why are obstetricians still the choice of most parents?

Although home birth will not become accepted medical practice any time soon, it has had an effect on hospital deliveries. An increasing number of hospitals are allowing physicians and midwives to practice various natural childbirth methods in birthing rooms and in delivery rooms. This has had and will continue to have a great impact on obstetrical patients in the future. The job of the home birth movement is not finished. It must continue to force doctors into recognizing that patients are intelligent human beings who can make a choice about medical care.

## Summary

There are numerous practices and procedures being used by obstetricians today that have dangerous implications: the use of electronic fetal monitors, elective induction of delivery, and the rising incidence of cesarean section. As the public is becoming more educated on the medical care issues, they are questioning the judgment of physicians more frequently. This has led to the demand for alternatives in health care. One alternative people are turning to is home childbirth.

The process of home birth involves a completely natural delivery by a trained midwife. There is absolutely no unnecessary intervention in the process. The woman delivers when she is ready, in the presence of her husband and family if she wishes, with no help from technical devices. This method has been shown to be as safe as, if not safer than, hospital delivery. Physicians still refuse to accept it as an alternative, however. This has caused a polarization between home birth advocates and physicians, which is detrimental to the physician-patient relationship.

There are many reasons physicians disapprove of home birth, among them because it challenges the authority of the physician and established medical practices, and because it is a threat to the earning power of physicians. Regardless of physician disapproval, however, mothers are turning to home birth because of the higher quality of deliveries associated with it. It has been determined that there is a misunderstanding between what physicians perceive as quality care, and how mothers view quality care. Most women who have experienced home birth agree that it is much more satisfying than that in the hospital. Home birth does not seem likely to be practiced on a large scale in the future, but it is receiving wider acceptance. A possible solution to the controversy is the implementation of home birth rooms in the hospital. The result would be the quality of home for the mother and the safety of the hospital. This type of setting is becoming more available as physicians are learning to be responsive to patients' needs and desires. It should be considered a victory for home birth advocates, and all patients who want to be treated as active participants in decisions affecting their health.

# 10

# UNDERSTANDING AGING PARENTS AND GRANDPARENTS

The issue of responsibility of the young for the care of their older family members has been treated differently depending on the time and the culture. Medieval church law dictated that children were accountable for the care of their parents. The idea that the community should assist the elderly person was first established in Elizabethan poor law. This assistance was supposed to be given only after the children had done what could be done, but the law never fully clarified the extent of what was to be expected from the offspring. Today, state laws concerning the question of family responsibility to older members remain inconsistent.

The concept of filial responsibility, the obligation of adults to meet their parents' needs, refers not only to law and custom, but also to general attitudes. An increasing number of contemporary parents and children are faced with the reality of this concept as a result of extended life expectancies. Preventive medicine and health education have greatly affected longevity. Twenty million people in the United States, approximately 10 percent of the population, are now sixty-five years or older. Almost ten million are over seventy-three and one million are over eighty-five. By the year 2000, it is estimated that 25 percent of the population will be over the age of sixty-five.[1] As the issue of care for the elderly has become more urgent, the problems surrounding this issue have become more numerous and complex.

Before the 1930s, caring for the aged sick and disabled posed no real problem. First, the people who fit into this category comprised only 4 percent of the population. Second, the cohesive, extended family structure was such that these members were included in the nucleus of the family, and the responsibility for their care was assumed without question. But with industrialization and urbanization, a new social system evolved with a greater emphasis on the separation of the married couple from the original family unit, liberation of women, and the value of youth.[2] Traditionally, the psychological support and physical care of the aged had been primarily the responsibility of the female members of the family. The change in the social role of women has affected their position as primary caregiver to the elderly family member. Not only has this change resulted in more opportunities for women to pursue careers outside the home, if they choose to do so, but for many women the increased availability of work outside the home has created obligations that compete with their duties toward their aging parents. In many instances, it is necessary for the woman to assume some of the financial responsibilities to keep the family functioning. Drawn away from the home to fulfill these responsibilities, the woman is no longer available to care for the sick, dependent elders.

Besides social changes that can impose problems for the care of the aging parents, emotional problems can also create constraints. Mc-Greehan and Warburton view aging as a developmental crisis for families. They define crisis as a "significant turning point caused by an emotional or physical episode that will result in change of family members." Other such developmental crises include marriages, births, and separation of children from home. These developmental crises usually demand a change in the reciprocal role relationships between family members. Margaret Blekner (1965) supports this view, postulating a developmental phase called "filial maturity." This phase usually occurs at a time in an adult child's life when he or she is between the ages of forty and fifty and can no longer look to his or her parents for help with emotional or financial problems. The parents, in fact, may need the child's aid.

The change that precipitates this developmental crisis can be dramatic or subtle. Until the time of crisis, the reciprocal role relationship between aging parents and their adult children had been relatively stable. Children were involved with their own personal and family concerns. Their parents may have been involved in their lives to some extent, e.g., family get-togethers, family business, etc. But for the most part, the parents were removed from the lives of their children. Then, ultimately, a traumatic or subtle shift occurs in this relationship. The change can be dramatic if the parent suffers from a heart ailment, stroke, or cancer. Or it may be subtle as the adult children slowly become aware of their aging parent's increasing physical problems or decreasing mental acuity. Whether the change is subtle or dramatic, it brings with it a gradual role reversal. This shift in roles is often a very difficult transition for family members to accept, even when they realize that this phase of life ultimately comes to everyone. "Everywhere the human cycle begins with the dependency of the young on those who are older, and usually ends with the dependency of the very old on those who are younger."[3]

The anxiety and conflict that usually accompany this transition are compounded by individual psychological problems of family members. It is difficult for adult children to think of parents as old and no longer able to take care of themselves. They may be unable to give up what remains of their belief as children that their parents are omnipotent and immortal. Unable to relinquish parental support, adult children may deny their parents' failing capabilities and expect them to continue in a role that they can no longer play. They may not be able to accept the fact that they must now assume the parental role with those who used to care for them. In addition to the transition in their role relationship with their parents, adult offspring might be shifting roles with their own children, who are becoming teenagers and adults. Adult children may also find it difficult to relate to their aging parents because they are reminded of their own limited time. The problems of aging that the parent is experiencing may cause problems of adjustment in the child. Adult children have to face the inevitability of a time when they too will be going through the process of aging and the possibility that they may become dependent upon their children for even their most basic needs.

Just as their adult children are having difficulty in accepting the changes that are occurring in their aging parents, the elders themselves may be unable to deal with these changes. Elderly parents may not be able to accept their declining capabilities and may deny these inevitable changes. Not wanting their children to find out about their difficulties, they may affect a facade of independence. The older persons may develop feelings of resentment against the young. They see in the young the attractiveness, vigor, and sexual prowess that they are lacking. Angry at the brevity of life, they may resent those who have before them the life span they have already completed.

An understanding by children and parents of the psychological stresses that both are suffering may help to smooth the transition. Many of the difficulties in adjustment that both young and old experience may be the result of a lack of communication, for the two generations see aging and its implications from different viewpoints. Before adult children can relate to their parents in a meaningful way, they must try to understand the deprivations and stresses that aging imposes. First, they must realize that the aged are at a period in life in which they have many more contacts with dying and death. The aged experience not only anticipatory grief over the death of self, but also bereavement at the continuous loss of personal relationships. Anticipatory grief may be the aged's reaction to the loss of social role, self-esteem, independence, a lifetime home, or the failure of bodily functions or sensory acuity. Elderly people who are grieving in anticipation over the threatened loss of self tend to begin withdrawing from life processes, partly as preparation for the acceptance of a lesser role in life. The family of the aged who is experiencing grief or bereavement may relate to the individual as if nothing were wrong. This pretense is assumed because the family believes that it will help the individual maintain his or her dignity and privacy. In reality, it denies the elderly person the opportunity to discuss certain immediate losses and the fear of future losses.

If adult children are aware of the losses that are experienced by their aging parents, they will be better able to understand their parents' outward expression of their reaction to these losses. Instead of seeing stubbornness as a burdensome trait of the old, the young should realize that this reaction may be a desperate attempt to hold onto lifestyles or remaining possessions. Instead of seeing their parents' withdrawal as a lack of feeling, adult children need to understand that isolation is a normal reaction to a painful loss. Repeated memories concerning persons in the elder's past should not be dismissed as senility, but should be seen as an expression of losses that have been included in the aged's grieving processes. The older family member may just now be grieving for the loss of a loved one who died many years ago. If children understand the underlying dynamics of their parents' behavior, they will not be so quick to take these reactions as failures on their own part.

Children must also realize that their aging parents' needs are very similar to those of the young. Besides the basic needs, the aged also need to feel useful, active, and independent. We sometimes act as if we believe that after a certain age an individual can no longer be expected to develop or to make any further contributions to society. Old age is not just a time in which an older person waits for death. If we view old age in this way, we stunt the later growth of the elderly and cause them to feel inferior and useless. This makes it difficult and frustrating for an older person to continue to live. Rather, we should adopt the attitude of the Abkhasians in the Soviet Union who describe their elders as "long living" rather than old.[4] The connotation of this term is one of continuing life rather than approaching death.

Adult children must allow aging parents to maintain some degree of control over their lives. One of the greatest issues confronting aged parents and their children is the question of whether to live together or separately. Both parents and children should be involved in making this decision. Much research suggests that many of the elderly do not want to move in with their children, preferring to keep their independence as long as possible. They would rather live in their own homes because this allows them to maintain their sense of autonomy. One elderly woman expressed this desire for independence as follows: "I don't want to be living with my kids. I love them. I don't want to have, you know, any misunderstandings. Why, if I were to live there, I couldn't have friends in so easy or cook on my stove. I have my friends and the kids have their friends. It's better all 'round just visiting and being close."[5] A recent national survey revealed that most elderly feel this reluctance to give up their independence; only 10 percent of the sample of old people expressed the desire to live with a child or relative.[6] Adult children do not always understand their parents' wish for independence. They worry about their parents living alone and try to persuade the elders to live with them. This is especially true in those instances when the death of a spouse leaves one parent alone. Children immediately assume that their parent would be better off moving out of his or her home, not realizing that the house might be a comfort to the grieving parent because of its familiarity and the good memories it holds.

Old people should be allowed to maintain their independence as long as they choose to do so or as long as they possibly can. Many community services are available to help the old maintain their independence. Homemakers can help the elderly manage their household, by working on their budget, housecleaning, and preparing meals. Through the Meals-on-Wheels programs, the aged may receive hot meals delivered by volunteers, who are usually also willing to visit with recipients for a short while. In addition, visiting nurses provide services for elderly persons who are unable to travel to a doctor's office. However, the physical limitations of the aged may become so incapacitating that these social services are not sufficient to allow the old person to remain at home. But the necessity for the old person to leave home is not always obvious or acceptable to the elderly. Home care should be strongly emphasized.

Elderly individuals may value their independence to such an extent that they cling to it even after they are no longer able to live by themselves. Many old people are reluctant to give up their independence because they are aware of society's disapproval of dependency in an adult. The aged are often reluctant to seek help despite their urgent need because they view their declining abilities and dependency as evidence of regression to a more childlike state. The elderly must face the loss of ability to perform such tasks as walking, writing, and control of elimination processes — tasks that were learned in the early years of development. The aged may feel anxiety about increased dependency and suffer from their own and society's disapproval.

Eventually, the declining capabilities of the elderly and their inability to live alone can no longer be denied by the aging parents or their adult children. Families are then confronted with the problem of how to care for aging members who can no longer care for themselves. They must decide on the new living arrangements for the aged person. Aging parents and adult children should decide whether the elder will live together with the family or separately in a nursing home or retirement community. Many factors should be considered before arriving at a suitable arrangement.

The adult children may experience ambivalent feelings when they are faced with the decision of either bringing their parents into their own home or finding another solution. They want to do everything possible for their parents, but they also want to keep disruption of their own life to a minimum. Remembering all that their parents have done for them, adult children may feel guilty for thinking of their parents as a burden or inconvenience. The aging begin to make self-accusations also. They feel that they should be grateful and happy to be asked to come to live with their offspring. But they fear that their status will be reduced to that of their children's children. Most important, parents and children must decide whether living together is within the scope of their physical and emotional capabilities. If the decision is made to incorporate the parent into the household, additional problems may arise.

Parents living with their children works well in some instances. This is particularly true when a close relationship between the generations has been maintained throughout the years of separate living. But many circumstances can make sharing living quarters difficult and sometimes even impossible. Crowded conditions in the home, financial worries, friction with in-laws, and ineffective communication are among a few of these trying conditions. An example of the latter occurs when the adult children are worried about making their parents feel inadequate and useless, but want them to live comfortably without the burdens of household responsibilities. At the same time, the parents may have the desire to be helpful and to "carry their share of the burden," but they do not want to interfere in the affairs of the household.

To help assuage the first two conditions mentioned, limited space and financial worries, society should offer more support systems. As of yet, there are few such support systems to help adults fulfill their obligations of filial responsibility. Respite services are available that provide families with occasional or systematic relief from arduous duties of caring for ill and disabled older members. Day care programs give respite to families who may need a place for an older family member to stay while children work. Home aides, Meals-on-Wheels, and dial-a-ride transportation are available to alleviate some of the burden from the primary-care person. But state and federal programs should also provide financial assistance to help families maintain their older members at home if they wish to do so. Loans and funds for construction of additions to homes should be available. *Governmental programs should also consider the wisdom of direct subsidies to families that participate in daily care of elderly relatives.* In a series of investigative articles in the *New York Times* concerning New York City nursing homes in 1974–75, John L. Hess pointed out that in the state of New York, Medicaid pays the staggering sum of $10,000 per bed per year to a nursing home. This money, which figures out to $833 a month, could be paid directly to families who care for an aged patient at home.[7] Families that overcome the many problems of home care of the elderly deserve these payments just as much as strangers who provide less personalized care. The concept of filial responsibility has implications for social policy as well as for individual and family adjustment. Government policy makers must decide whether to support adults' obligations to care for their aging parents or to further develop governmental and community services.

Social support services and programs such as these might mean an increase in the family's ability to maintain an important relationship with an aging member. They might allow a family to fulfill their filial obligations to an aging member. But no matter what social services and programs are provided, they can supplement but not substitute for the emotional bonds between aging parents and adult children.

Many of the aged's dependent needs can be and usually are met by their family members. Relatives substitute their strength, mobility, and judgment for the old person's declining abilities. But there may come a time when the family is no longer able to meet the needs of the elder. Care of the aging parents can become an excessive burden, overwhelming the family to the point that it endangers the physical, emotional, and social stability of its members. At this point, the need for separate living arrangements must be accepted by both parties. Institutionalization, in these cases, is not necessarily a matter of callous indifference on the part of the children, but rather a last resort taken after prolonged hesitation and after other alternatives have been tried and found wanting.

A primary reason given for putting an old person in a nursing home is that it is "best for the parent." In cases where living together has been tried and is no longer possible, this is a rational explanation for putting an aged family member in an institution. The elderly parent may be senile or have other physical, mental, or emotional problems that require specialized care family members cannot provide. Other times this reason is just a rationalization, an attempt by the adult child to reduce the anxiety caused by feelings of guilt. Some children may find it "inconvenient" or impractical for the aging parent to live in their home. Fortunately, this is most often not the case. Usually the institutionalization of parents for appropriate reasons, when relocation in a nursing home is truly "best for the parent," is an easier separation for both parties to accept. Mentally healthy parents will be better able to understand the need for the separation, with the acceptance of their limitations. Disoriented parents may have a more difficult time, experiencing confusion and helplessness. Both healthy and disoriented parents will still react to the move to a nursing home with grief and loss.

The relocation of aged family members to a nursing home is a trying adjustment for both parents and children. The aged often associate this move with loss of independence, optimal physical capability, friends, personal belongings, and control. In addition, the elderly may experience feelings of rejection, anger, abandonment, and apprehension. The family also may feel guilt about "putting away" an older family member into a nursing home, fear of criticism, and anger for having to make such an uncomfortable decision.

Death is often associated with nursing homes in the minds of both aging parents and adult children. It has been estimated that some 80 percent of the aged do eventually end up dying in institutions rather than in their own home. Thus the need for home care. Because nursing homes are often thought of as "houses of death," both parents and children fear them. For many families, admission to an old people's home is so symbolic of death that they either openly or subtly grieve for a person as though he or she were already dead. Because the institution is a painful reminder of death, family members are tempted to visit the elder relative less and less frequently. Both families and institutionalized patients need help in dealing with their reactions to nursing homes so that the family relationship can be maintained to the greatest extent possible. Frequent visits by adult children will help family members maintain the strong emotional bond that is so important to the psychological, physical, and emotional health of all involved. Visits can sometimes lose their positive value and become strained for both children and parents. Some children are uncomfortable about visiting their aged parents in nursing homes. A typical complaint is "there is nothing to do; we just sit there."[8] They fail to realize that they might be supporting their parents emotionally just by their presence and interest in their welfare. If these visits are relaxed and informal, and meaningful communication is maintained, the relationship between aged parents and adult children can continue to be rewarding. Adult children must not be afraid to bring their own children to visit their grandparents in a nursing home. If they try to protect their young children from the nursing home situation, the youngsters will not have the opportunity to engage in meaningful contact with their grandparents.

As their parents go through the process of aging, adult children must understand the deprivations and stresses that aging imposes. In this way both the aging parent and the adult child will be better able to accept the developmental phase of aging and its implications. Family members must recognize the value of the older member as an individual who has the ability to make a meaningful contribution to the family, regardless of his or her frailty and dependence. Too often the young do not realize that they can learn much from the old. Adult children and grandchildren can obtain valuable information and insight by listening to older family members' stories of the past. Sophocles expressed the instructive benefits of "conversing" with the old in Plato's *Dialogues*: "There is nothing I like better, Cephalus, than conversing with aged men; for I regard them as travellers who have gone a journey which I too may have to go, and of whom I ought to inquire whether the way is smooth and easy, or rugged and difficult."[9]

From their aged parents children can gain a better understanding of the forces that shaped their parents' lives and have, in turn, influenced their own development. More important, adult children will be better prepared to face their own aging process and the "hands in their future" will not feel as cold and unfamiliar.

# 11

# HOME CARE FOR THE ELDERLY: AN ALTERNATIVE TO INSTITUTIONALIZATION

Current information about alternatives to institutional care of the aged is inadequate to use as a basis for changing public policy. Because so many of the aged are institutionalized unnecessarily, however, the importance of restructuring the financing and organization of care must be stressed.

This chapter will address both the need and the potential for creating a new system of care for the elderly that will use society's scarce resources wisely and efficiently.

There are many unmet needs among the elderly, and the problem is growing. The population aged sixty-five and over is on the increase, due to a reduced birth rate and greater longevity. Especially dramatic is the rise in the numbers and proportions of people aged seventy-five and over—an age when individuals are more likely to be ill than those aged sixty-five to seventy-four. Retirement or the loss of a supporter or companion often leaves many elderly people with inadequate resources, thus making them dependent on their families or, in many cases, on society. The question is, will society care enough to commit adequate resources to long-term care? Most attention to long-term care has been focused on institutional care, with very little thought given to alternative approaches. There are, however, hopeful signs. As the elderly become an increasingly important group numerically, they also become increasingly important politically. As political power is harnessed and directed, this group is bound to gain attention.

Concerns about the costs and limits of Medicare and Medicaid, about the appropriateness and the quality of the care provided in nursing homes, and about the negative and dehumanizing effects of long-term institutionalization have led to an interest in alternatives. The private sector, represented by such third-party payers as Blue Cross, has become interested in the potential cost savings of alternative programs and has become involved in the funding of home care. Fifty-two of the nation's sixty-nine Blue Cross plans now offer some type of home health care coverage. More than forty-two million Blue Cross Plan subscribers have such coverage.[1]

Much of the interest in alternatives arises from the potential for cost savings. But, regardless of cost, there is general agreement that the effectiveness of a long-term care system is partly dependent on its ability to provide a continuum of care, the continuum being, on one end, community support services that would enable a minimally impaired person to live independently. Such services include in-home care, such as homemaker services and Meals-on-Wheels, and out-of-home services, such as senior citizen centers and day care. On the other end of the continuum are the institutions for the elderly where the ill, disabled, or mentally impaired elderly can receive skilled nursing care. In between these two extremes there exist congregate and sheltered housing for those who do not require extensive personal care services but who have difficulty managing in their own homes.

The present health and social service system in the United States has not come close to reaching this continuum. Too many elderly people are placed in institutions, not for medical reasons, but because the resources needed to sustain them in their homes are lacking. For example, in Massachusetts it was found that only thirty-seven percent of the one hundred thousand patients in licensed nursing homes required full-time nursing care, and fourteen percent needed no institutional care at all. Similar situations were also reported elsewhere.[2]

Not only is this problem costly to society, but the needs of the aged are not being met. In order to alleviate the problem, alternatives must exist; and this is where the difficulty lies. Very little information exists on alternatives and their success, while at the same time these alternatives must provide care for the elderly at least at the existing level and at no higher cost to the individual or to society.

As the system exists now, several key problems have been identi-

fied: inadequate coordination, limited alternatives to institutionalization, frustrating bureaucratic maze, and limited income.³

The services of many agencies and institutions concerned with
health and social problems of the elderly are inadequately coordinated. These organizations often function well independently, but
they tend to interact only when required to do so by regulation or
necessity. This shortcoming is particularly evident in the lack of communication between health and social service organizations regarding each other's capabilities.

Because Medicare, Medicaid, and private programs tend to reimburse institutional care more readily than home care, and because
few communities have adequate home care services, elderly people
are often institutionalized when home care programs would be more
appropriate. This can cause a problem for the institution as well as
for the elderly person, because the institution may have to refuse admission to some patients who need such care if no space is available.

In seeking appropriate services or support from local or state organizations, the elderly person may be confronted with a frustrating
maze of office locations, applications, and financial requirements.
Limited capacity to cope with these frustrations may be enough to
discourage further action by the elderly person.

The elderly person's limited income, coupled with restricted third-
party benefits, may necessitate accepting only those services that are
reimbursed. Similarly, limited protection by public and private third
parties in terms of types and quantities of services and dollar payments
can inhibit any health care provider in the attempt to deliver appropriate care.

Since institutions seem to be an inappropriate setting for at least
some of the elderly they serve, and since they are unable to provide
for all the needs of the impaired elderly, alternatives such as day care
and home care must be developed.

The development of geriatric day care programs in the United
States is in the experimental stages. Unlike Britain, where day hospitals and day care centers are well developed and have distinct places
in the health and social services system, here in the United States very
few geriatric day care centers exist.⁴ The federal government defines
day care as "a program of services provided under health leadership
in an ambulatory setting for adults who do not require 24-hour institutional care and yet, because of physical or mental impairment, are

not capable of full-time independent living. Day hospitals and day-care services provide protective environments with therapeutic programs for the impoverished elderly."[5] The main goal of geriatric day care should be to prevent or delay institutionalization by maintaining people in the community.

Two types of patients are generally accommodated in day care centers. The first type requires long-term care. In this case, day care provides an alternative to institutionalization. The second type of patient needs day care as a short-term transition from an acute hospital or long-term institution to more independent living.[6]

Another alternative to institutional care is home care. Basically, home care refers to the provision of skilled nursing services within the home. The American Medical Association defines home care as "any arrangement for providing, under medical supervision, needed health care and supportive services to a sick or disabled person in his/her home surroundings."

In the United States, however, home care receives a very low priority. Although home care is provided under both Medicare and Medicaid, expenditures for home health care constitute less than 1 percent of either budget.[7]

Overall, health care professionals in the private sector have not contributed significantly to developing or increasing home care programs. There are several factors that may contribute to this. For example, professional attitudes and behavior tend to encourage institutionalization. Because the range of services generally available from home health agencies is limited, physicians are often reluctant to place patients in the home situation, where there is a danger of regression due to lack of needed care. Physicians also tend to prefer the relative efficiency with which patients can be treated in nursing homes and hospitals. However, efficiency seems to be considered from the point of view of the physician's time, rather than in terms of efficiency in the delivery of health services. Another factor might be that inpatients who require little medical attention are profitable customers. Often, hospitals with low capacity are reluctant to part with such patients. Although this unprofessional attitude may have its basis in a societal orientation toward institutionalization, the wishes of families who would prefer to support a relative at home, if appropriate resources were available to them, must be respected.

Appropriate funding, then, seems to be a major stumbling block to alternative methods of care. For instance, Medicare focuses on acute or short-term illness by requiring prior hospitalization of at least three days, by limiting the number of visits by personnel in the home health agency to one hundred per year, and by paying for only "skilled care." The Medicare requirement of "skilled care" restricts reimbursement mainly to services provided by relatively highly trained professionals, such as nurses, physical therapists, and speech pathologists. Under Medicare, the patient must be evaluated as needing the services of at least one of these professionals to be eligible for reimbursement of other home health services. This requirement persists even though it has been shown that homemaker–home health aide and such related support services as meals and transportation can be equally as important as the "skilled" services in maintaining the elderly person at home and in preventing needless institutionalization. Thus a major problem with the Medicare system is that the home health services that are reimbursable are not those that are most needed by the majority of the insured group; medical services are emphasized, whereas many needed social services are ignored. There are problems with Medicaid coverage of home care as well. Current Medicaid regulations mandate all states to provide nursing and home health aide services, as well as medical supplies and equipment. But Medicaid, too, fails to cover the multiplicity of services required of a comprehensive home care program. Also, although federal guidelines do not limit the number of visits an eligible person may receive, individual states are allowed to impose such limitations.

The development of home health care has also been impeded by insurance company policies. Until recently, hardly any insurance companies included home health benefits as part of their medical coverage.

In addition to problems of financing, lack of coordination between various agencies has also caused problems for a home care program. Separate services offered by a multitude of agencies are often confusing to the public. When unfamiliar with the variety of services available and the procedures for obtaining them, the process seems long and difficult. Usually decisions need to be made quickly and services are needed immediately. Unless knowledgeable help is given, institutionalization seems like a simple and quick solution.

Finally, there is the program of availability. Present funding programs have no built-in strategy to ensure that care is equally available to all who are in need. It is no help to an individual that Medicare pays for home care services if in his or her community such services do not exist. Furthermore, in some locations, particularly rural areas and inner cities, there are no home health services at all. In rural areas, lack of transportation can also cause problems, because even those scarce services that exist are inaccessible to many persons.

Despite the problems, there has been a growing interest in alternatives to institutionalization, especially in day care and home care, by government, consumers, third-party payers, and professionals. A major reason for this interest is the widespread belief in the cost-effectiveness of noninstitutional care. Savings result when the availability of alternatives either prevents institutionalization or allows earlier discharge. Effectiveness is seen in the potential for alternative programs to improve health care, functioning abilities, independence, and life satisfaction of the elderly.

The number of elderly people in need of services is expected to rise significantly in the future. As demand for services increases, expenditures for them will be stimulated by the growth of the elderly population and by the expanded services that will become available to the elderly. This increased demand should stimulate the analysis of alternatives, and of their potential for effectiveness relative to cost, in comparison with the present system.

I have mentioned several problems and inadequacies of the health care system as it now exists in the United States. Institutions are not always appropriate and options such as day care and home care should be part of a spectrum of alternatives designed so that choices are based on what is good for the patient and what is reasonable for the payer.

Major changes must be made in our current health care system if the elderly population is to be appropriately cared for. First, Medicare and Medicaid must be amended so that their coverage includes an adequate array of noninstitutional services. Second, we must introduce and fund with public money agencies for the elderly that would operate on a community basis and provide such services as day care and home care, as needed. These agencies should be staffed with teams trained to deal with the total patient—such as a nurse and a social worker—teams that can address the patient's social as well as medical needs. The main objective should be to provide a system that offers enough choice so that services appropriate to individual patient needs can be provided.

# 12

## A NEW LOOK AT
## HOME CARE FOR THE AGED

A ging is characterized by the concurrence of multiple dysfunctions. Elderly persons (sixty-five years and older) are more likely to suffer from chronic disease and the resultant disability. These same individuals also are increasingly vulnerable to social, psychological, and economic stresses. The aged and homebound people are among the medically unreached. They are out of contact with the medical care system because they are often impoverished and too disabled, frightened, or bewildered to reach out. Nor does assistance usually go to them. Our inability to provide good health care for the rapidly growing number of older persons in our society is becoming a problem of great national concern. The high cost of health care is likely to be driven still higher by the need to serve this growing population, already the leading consumers of health care. The problem is complicated by the nature of our health care system. Philip W. Brickner, M.D., suggests the elderly can be helped only through the development of comprehensive programs that provide services in the home.

Home care is a program of integration between doctors, nurses, and social workers. These teams must be based in hospitals, with the full support of a consultative staff that is willing to go to the home if needed. Home health care of the aged is a combined hospital-community responsibility. The potential for broad, community-based home health programs capable of serving large population groups with varying and fluctuating needs has barely been demonstrated. Hospital-based programs are also in short supply and are not being developed in proportion to their need. Home health services, where they do exist, are underfinanced, limited in their capacity to cover the population in need. Generally, home health services for the older person have been limited by the short supply of programs and do not provide more than the "nursing plus one" services. What is needed is an overall federal policy for home health care. Home health care programs will succeed only if there is clarity of purpose and method. Goals must be established that express the needs of both the patients and members of the staff, and the community at large must perceive that the general good is being served. Dr. Brickner reveals three goals for home care for the aged: (1) for the patients, staying out of institutions, in their homes, with maximum independence; (2) for the staff, professional fulfillment and personal satisfaction; (3) for the community, helping families stay together, decreasing the number of patients in nursing homes, and saving public money. These goals must be directed toward the needs of real people, and planning must be for the long term.[1] Why is home care for the aged crucial?

Older people are at a pivotal moment in their lives. Living alone, they may be able for a while to sustain an independent life, exist in safety, obtain food, keep clean. But any small change in their condition (state of health) will create a downward spiral. A bad state of health will restrict activity, cause poor nourishment, confusion and panic, deterioration of living quarters, physical and intellectual failure. Often older people are unable to reach out for help — they know no one, cannot get assistance on the telephone, are ignored. Deterioration increases, and institutionalization may become inevitable, often resulting in death. If comprehensive medical and social services are provided in the home at the right moment, an independent life can be sustained. Home health services often prevent or delay transfer from the home.

The physical characteristics of advanced age are common knowledge: loss of hair and teeth, feebleness, poor recent memory, failure of hearing and vision. The elderly are a heterogeneous part of the population, with diverse needs and capacities. The proportion of elderly people in the United States has increased, due to the high fertility rate in the late nineteenth century to the mid-twentieth century and the general decrease in the birth rate. Those who were part of the baby boom that followed World War II will join the over-sixty-five population after 2010, causing rapid expansion of this age group.

Under current laws, home health care is supported primarily

under Medicare, Medicaid, Title XX, and the Older Americans Act. Differing eligibility requirements, services, and responsibilities for research, demonstrations, and evaluation create a sense of underlying confusion in the administration of home care programs.[2] In January 1975, there were approximately 2,247 certified home health agencies in the United States (National League for Nursing, 1975). Some home care programs are sponsored by public health departments or receive community support through the United Way or other fund-raising efforts. Services are provided through so many different programs that effective coordination and delivery of home health and other in-home services seems close to impossible. For this reason there needs to be a program in which services would be provided through a single entry point. Theodore Koff (1982) suggests coordinated services, centralized intake, and case management. This model can be a solution to the multitude of programs currently being implemented. Adult day health services, senior centers, housing, nutrition services, and homemaker services are some programs that are accessible to older persons. These programs are adequate for some of the aged, but the system does not locate the frail older person living alone. Most important, these programs are not properly funded and are not integrated into one system, therefore proper assessment is not assured. A system needs to be coordinated that would be accessible not only to the easy to reach, but also to the isolated. This would establish a well-integrated, controlled system, which would ensure proper assessment, monitoring, and funding and would enrich the quality of life of the older person.

## Adult Day Health Services

Adult day health services are not a single service but a range of services provided in a variety of settings.

Day care services are defined as:

> Services whereby patients are transported, often in specially equipped vehicles, to a common setting for purposes of receiving medical-nursing and health-related social services with the aim of helping them attain physical rehabilitation or maintain their current physical status. Patients may spend from several hours in the day care facility for a period of one to five days a week. Day

care may be provided under the auspices of a hospital, nursing home or extended care facility. The services of the day care facility are often merged with the operation of the sponsoring facility and usually include physical therapy, group therapy, occupational therapy, speech therapy, specific nursing procedures, dentistry, podiatry, and personal care. The aim of day care services is to dissociate the "hotel" element of hospital care from therapeutic content, leaving only the latter.[3]

Participants in adult day health interventions assist in rehabilitation or restorative activities. Some early programs still functioning are the Adult Day Treatment Center, established under private auspices in 1965 in Beverly Hills, California; the Mansfield Home in Mansfield, Ohio; and St. Otto's Nursing Home Day Care Program, which was opened in 1969 and became the first "subacute care" facility in New York State to be licensed for outpatient services. Today there are an estimated six hundred such programs. Unfortunately, consistent funding and licensing or certifying criteria are absent from these programs and hinder the development of high standards and the expansion of this important service.

Programs are funded through Titles XVIII, XIV, and XX of the Social Security Act, the Older Americans Act, revenue sharing, United Way, and direct payments by participants.

## Senior Centers

Senior centers, in contrast to the adult day health services, serve as places where older persons can meet, receive services, and participate in activities that will enhance their dignity, support their independence, and encourage their involvement in and with the community. They build upon the social functioning of older people. Senior centers respond to the needs of older persons able to participate in a self-directing program.

The William Hodson Community, established in 1943, was the first senior center. A recent (1974) directory of senior centers lists nearly five thousand clubs and senior centers in the United States. The growth of centers closely corresponds to the flow of federal dollars made available to senior centers after passage of the 1965 Older Americans Act.

## Housing

Of all the problems that homebound, aged people face, the most difficult to solve is the need for adequate housing. The Housing Act of 1965 authorized the construction of new housing (or remodeling of existing housing) specifically designed for elderly families.

The Congregate Housing Services Act of 1978 promoted the coordination of supportive services, maintaining independence for those temporarily disabled or handicapped. This type of housing provides an environment that encourages older persons to be as independent as possible. It enables them to remain outside institutional environments, which provide more intensive medical services.

In New York City, half of the households headed by persons over age sixty-five have a yearly income of $3,000 or less. Rent control was established to help the elderly by limiting the amount of rent they have to pay. It has enabled many aged people to remain in their own apartments. In New York, the state rent control law has been of significant value. Many aged people in New York City occupy relatively inexpensive housing units and have been in the same place for years. Although this program helps the elderly stay at home, many tenants have complained that they have been harassed and denied building services by landlords who wanted them to move. Recent attempts to modify the law have focused on controlled rents only for people in genuine financial need.[4]

Congregate housing and rent control are just two programs intended to minimize the housing problem. They can be considered home care services because they try to accommodate the older person's needs, and one of these needs is to stay home. But the needs of the elderly cannot be met by housing alone; housing must be accompanied by appropriate services. Housing for the elderly should be developed with or in proximity to senior centers, nutrition programs, and other health-related services so that these services are accessible.

## Food and Nutrition

Elderly people commonly have difficulty organizing a proper nutritional program for themselves. It is not easy to sustain interest in preparing and eating meal after meal alone. The elderly have special nutritional problems, because they have special health, educational, economic, transportation, and sociological problems.[5]

Poverty, physical disability, and lack of knowledge and skill are three problems that affect one's access to food and one's diet. Almost a third of people over age sixty-five in the United States live on an income of less than $4,000 a year.[6] Many aged individuals who survive on public assistance and Social Security find they have no money left at the end of the month to purchase food, and for reasons of pride or ignorance they will not publicly acknowledge their poverty to social workers or others who might help them.

People of advanced age often suffer from physical disability, which can interfere with their ability to obtain or prepare food. Arthritis, failing vision, or mental confusion can make shopping seem too much of an effort, and even such simple procedures as opening cans, taking off cellophane wrappers, opening screw-top bottles, peeling potatoes, and slicing bread can present real problems to the frail, older person.[7]

Inadequate information about nutritional value and inexperience with cooking techniques are common difficulties that interfere with the maintenance of a proper diet for older people. Lack of motivation tempts the elderly to select foods that require little preparation and are of low nutritional value. Older people, like their younger counterparts, often are simply ignorant about what constitutes a good diet. Attempts to solve this problem center around the home delivery of meals to those people who cannot leave home and group meal programs that serve individuals who are less handicapped.

## Meals-on-Wheels Program

The delivery of food to the person in need is a key factor in the success of a home health care program for the aged. Meals-on-Wheels programs are based throughout the country and are made possible by Titles III, IV, and VII of the Older Americans Act of 1965.[8] It was not until the 1973 Comprehensive Service Amendments to the Older Americans Act that federal policy provided funding for nutritional services for the aging. These programs are sponsored by a wide variety of voluntary and civic associations (women's clubs, community councils, and family service organizations) and professional nonprofit groups, such as the Visiting Nurse Service and hospital auxiliaries. Most programs operate Monday through Friday and deliver either one or two meals a day per person. Efforts are made, through the use of insulating and packaging techniques, to control the temperature of the food until it is delivered. The recipient is expected to heat it at the right time, or it may be designed to be eaten uncooked. Most Meals-on-Wheels programs rely on volunteers who use their own cars or public transportation to deliver meals.

Nutrition programs create a daily opportunity to oversee the client's home situation and to see that alternate home services are made available if the individual cannot come to the nutrition site. One advantage of these programs is that a planned approach to preventive health care can be established at nutrition sites. Those served can be made aware of their own needs met, and of the services available for doing so. The nutrition site and its related programs provide a valuable opportunity to assess the needs of the older person.

## Homemaker Services

The ultimate purpose of the homemaker is to help patients meet home health and social needs. Homemakers work under the supervision of professional members of the health team. The homemaker is the eyes and ears of the team, able to report on patient status when others are not present, at the same time performing domestic chores and personal and paraprofessional duties. The homemaker sees the patient more frequently than any other member of the health care team and therefore is in the best position to note changes. The ability of this person to report changes in the patient's condition to the professional health team can be of critical value.

A system of organization for this growing form of service has not been established yet. One-fourth of known homemaker programs are independent.[9] There is no national standard of quality, but an attempt at creating guidelines is being made by the National Council for Homemaker Home Health Aide Services. Homemaker service agencies, whether public or voluntary, independent or a suborganization within a larger agency, seek financial support from a variety of resources, mostly from public tax monies and federal government funds supplied through the states. Funds from the federal government come through grants from various governmental departments, including the Department of Health, Education, and Welfare, the Welfare Administration, the Bureau of Family Services, the Children's Bureau, and the United States Public Health Service.

People employed in this program are engaged in services related to the health, safety, and general welfare of their aged clients. Specific functions include domestic chores, personal care, and paraprofessional health care. Often the elderly simply lack the strength, energy, and agility necessary to clean the house, do the laundry, and prepare meals. In most cases there is no family member or friend to step in and help. Domestic chores usually include preparing and serving meals; making and changing beds; dusting and vacuuming; dishwashing; tidying the kitchen, bathroom, and bedroom; listing needed supplies; shopping for supplies and doing errands; doing the client's personal laundry, ironing, and mending; emptying the garbage; cleaning and defrosting the refrigerator; reading and writing for the patient; and paying bills. Personal care tasks generally include care of teeth and mouth; grooming; care of the hair; shaving; care of the nails; bathing; helping the patient on and off the bedpan, commode, or toilet; moving from bed to chair or wheelchair; walking, dressing, and exercising; preparing and serving meals on diets prescribed by the physician. Paraprofessional health care is that which requires training and supervision of the homemaker by the physician or nurse responsible for the patient. Some routine health care tasks include back rubs, exercises, massages, help in use of support devices, observation and keeping records of important signs (temperature, pulse, and respiration), irrigation of Foley catheter, assistance with change of colostomy bag, administration of medication. For many older people the homemaker is the only human being they see. She can reduce the patient's isolation and can also maintain morale and possibly help avert depression.[10]

Despite these accomplishments, however, we still have no comprehensive, coordinated national policy on aging. Our nation has addressed the needs of older people in small increments, and this has created a fragmented and uncoordinated series of systems by which to meet these needs. Not only has this fragmentation led to the creation of a plethora of governmental agencies with different regulations, varied eligibility criteria, and separate administrative authorities, but it has also worked against the development of comprehensive, integrated, and effective service delivery to older people in their local communities.[11] The Administration on Aging, the state units, and the area agencies have not been given adequate funding or authority to carry out their responsibilities. Many of the elderly have done or are doing poorly. The challenge ahead is to work actively to bring out services and those of other systems closer together, to engage in more comprehensive and coordinated planning for the elderly, and to mesh more effective services from different systems to benefit individuals.

## Alternative Home Care Models

The aging are destined to become a larger and more influential segment of Amercian society. The falling birth rate, beginning in the early 1960s, coupled with increases in life expectancy, makes this demographic shift inevitable. The aging of the United States increasingly face negative influences, including loss of prestige, reduced opportunity for gainful employment, and declining family contact. Between 2010 and 2020, a net increase of approximately nine million persons is projected, an increase that is as large as the entire aging population in the United States as of 1940.[12] The proportion of the over-sixty-five population that is also seventy-five or older is increasing.

John M. Dobbin (1983) suggests that the need for alternative methods of providing health care and treatment for senior citizens is evident because of three major factors: the overall life span of senior citizens is lengthening, long-term care residents may be affected by constant moving to various facilities, and construction and operation costs for health care facilities are escalating. Dobbin suggests an alternative method in which individuals coming from their private residences would be able and willing to pay $45,000 in cash for their future care for the rest of their life beyond the ten-year period. This amount, times 150 residents, totals $6,575,000, which would be adequate to construct a 150-bed facility debt free. This facility would provide three levels of care: lodge, nursing home, and auxiliary hospital. Each patient would be assessed by the nursing staff on a weekly basis to determine what level of care is required, and the government would reimburse the facility accordingly, based on a predetermined rate. Dobbin feels this method would permit the patient to receive the most appropriate care and allow for family participation. Although this model seems of reasonable value, it does not address the elderly who are poor or do not own a home.

Theodore Koff suggests the integrated home and service center model, whereby the elderly can continue in their own households, with the familiarity, convenience, security, and related neighbor social structure, if these resources are available. The service center is not viewed separately from the home, but is integrated within the network, which includes information, referral, outreach, multidisciplinary assessment centers, and case management. This would provide a single entry point, in order for the individual to be properly assessed of his or her needs, and once proper assessment is established the individual would be monitored. The service center must be nearby and convenient to residences. They may be senior centers, nutrition sites, health centers, private practitioners' offices, or any other organization providing these services. Koff feels this system would serve as an aid to the family. It would help provide care to the elderly person and would also teach the family to understand the changing functioning of the older person so they can participate effectively in appropriate care. Most services are delivered outside the home. There must be a close relationship between a service agency and the individual in need of services. This model offers the greatest opportunity for independence while the individuals' changing needs can be monitored through regular participation in the service program.

The integrated home and service center model provides:

1. primary setting in which services are offered — senior center or other health or recreational program
2. services:
   transportation
   meals
   health screening and clinics
   recreation
   education
   hobbies
   counseling
   physical exercise
   social and community action
   employment
   home chore services
   home health care
   housing renovation
   legal services
   telephone reassurance
   shopping assistance[13]

Few elderly people want to go to a nursing home. To help them retain their independence and quality of life, home health has its advantages. For example, they can adapt better at home; the home has been a part of their lives for a long time; memories from home are hard to replace. People generally prefer to live in their own homes, not in institutions. Many positive factors are involved in this preference. Home health can also prevent certain hazards of hospitalization, such as confusion, disorientation, infection, falls, personality conflicts, anxiety, and noise. Many observers and participants of home care programs contend that any service that keeps people out of hospitals and nursing homes has to save money and improve the quality of life for the patient. Home health care has many benefits that meet the needs of the elderly, but increasing these services will not insure cost reductions. Although the General Accounting Office agreed that home care increased elderly longevity and life satisfaction, it did not decrease hospital or nursing home utilization. Home health care clearly will not solve all of today's problems, but an effective home health program in the future may prevent many elderly from having to go into hospitals and institutions.[14]

Current home health care programs suffer from many problems, most stemming from the fact that they're not integrated within one system. They are just a conglomerate of systems that serve different needs for different groups of the elderly. Adult day health services focus on a population that is specifically in need of such health interventions as rehabilitation or restorative activities. Senior centers concentrate on those elderly who can meet at the center. Housing programs do not serve any particular population. Food and nutrition services and homemaker services focus on those who are homebound. This fragmentation may be the reason why home health care is not saving money. Cost savings could be achieved if eligibility for home health is tightly controlled and a specific population is selected to receive services.

Our current fee-for-service system encourages hospitalization. Changes will come when America moves away from hospital to home care. Dr. Lawson, a professor at the University of Connecticut Department of Community Medicine and Health Care, stressed greater physician education about alternative services. Fear of intrusion has kept some doctors from using home care. Doctors should accept alternative community resources. Whether or not doctors will allow "competition" with a home agency is yet to be seen. Competition may be reduced if home health agencies include doctors in an efficient way. More studies must be conducted in the following areas: new reimbursement schemes, greater physician education, and targeting of those eligible for programs.

The elderly population is a diverse group. There needs to be a single point of entry in which the elderly in need can be properly assessed and monitored. For those who can retain their quality of life to some degree, Theodore Koff's model would provide for their needs. The country would benefit because there would be less need for hospitalization, and thus less cost. But we need to look beyond costs. Changing values and attitudes are just as important. Alternatives to the current system are there; society and especially those involved in health care need to study and implement some of them.

Care of the elderly disabled relative is a responsibility that many families cannot bear on a continuous long-term basis, but there is an alternative. Respite care provides planned, intermittent, short-term care as periodic relief to the family and the caregivers responsible for twenty-four-hour continuous care of a frail family member. It also may preclude the need for institutionalization. The frail older person can stay in the community and avoid the dehumanizing environment of the institution. Family support plays a big role in this program; studies show 80 percent of the necessary support is offered by the family. Support programs and services for families who provide home health care to their chronically ill or disabled family member should be developed. A trained volunteer may come in for short periods of daytime relief for the caregiver. Respite care can be a powerful mechanism for supporting meaningful community life in old age. The high economic cost of institutionalization, the belief that community living best supports the quality of life in old age, and the realization that it is the family unit that is, in fact, the major health care provider for the elderly are all factors that have nudged health planners and providers toward the exploration of respite care.

Home services should be a right, not a privilege. For those elders who need more than the basic home service, respite care can be offered. The family, together with professional respite care workers, can increase the quality of life for the older person.

Changes in our present policy must be considered. The baby boom population, which will reach age sixty-five by the year 2010, is projected to increase the aged population by nine million persons. Our whole society is aging. Life expectancy continues to increase, as does the difference in life expectancy between men and women. An effective home health program also needs to be considered because the elderly of the future will be better educated and in better health than those of today. Policy changes need to start with doctors and integration of programs and agencies. If all the available programs come under one system, tight control and administration can be established. Attitudes toward our elderly also need to change. Staying out of institutions, professional fulfillment and satisfaction, helping families stay together, and saving public money are goals that we must work toward.

Home health care services provide older persons with the option to spend the rest of their years in a quality lifestyle. Hospitals and institutions can inhibit the quality of life. Most older people can live independently. With a little help and support, the idea of getting old will not be viewed negatively. Helping older people early will mean they will be less dependent upon public support over long periods of time and therefore will be less costly to society. The number of days of illness can be reduced through early prevention. We as a society need to offset the ill effects of this period of life with rehabilitative, restorative, and other ameliorative interventions.

# 13

## GROUP HOMES
## FOR THE AGED

The predicted rise in the next twenty years of the percentage of our population aged seventy-five and over will cause great demands on our group health care service. In today's society, there are several options for care of the older generation. Institutions, which include hospitals and nursing homes, private home care, and a new innovation, group homes, are among the most utilized. Group homes are able to focus on the psychological needs of this age group, as well as their physical, social, and environmental needs.

One of the major questions one can ask about group homes is "Who are the people in these homes?" They are predominantly very old, with the mean age eighty years. According to 1981 figures, 71 percent of the people in old age homes were over seventy-five. Also, there were many more women in group homes than there were men. There are several possible explanations for this, chief of which is that the life span of women is seven years longer than that of men. Obviously, this means more women are alone at an older age. Another reason is that the females in this age bracket did not lead a self-sufficient life when they were younger; women stayed home with their children and did not have to work for a living. Also older men tend to care for their spouses while they are still alive. The proportion of elderly women in the community was lower by 66 percent than those in old-age homes.[1] The marital status of these individuals proved quite interesting. The majority of the widowed or single persons of this age bracket were in old-age homes. Sixty-four percent of patients in old-age homes made a poor adjustment to the death of their marital partner, compared to only 10 percent in the community. This supports findings that difficulties coping with life were generally more manifest in old-age home groups.[2] Table 1 illustrates this.

**TABLE 1**
**Sex, Age and Marital Status[3]**

|  | sex | | age group | | | | marital status | | | |
|---|---|---|---|---|---|---|---|---|---|---|
|  | *m* | *f* | *70–74* | *75–79* | *80–84* | *85–89* | *M* | *S* | *D* | *W* |
| community | 34 | 66 | 29 | 15 | 9 | 7 | 41 | 10 | 5 | 44 |
| hospital | 35 | 65 | 28 | 20 | 7 | 4 | 41 | 11 | 9 | 39 |
| old-age home | 21 | 79 | 18 | 24 | 26 | 21 | 12 | 18 | 5 | 65 |

There was no significant difference in location and educational attainment among the residents of group homes. But, as Table 2 demonstrates, the previous occupation of elderly residents proved that the better the career, the more apt a person is to become a resident of an old-age home.

**TABLE 2**
**Education and Occupation[4]**

|  | education | | | | |
|---|---|---|---|---|---|
|  |  |  |  | technical college | university |
|  | *2–5* | *6–7* | *8–10* |  |  |
| community | 7 | 34 | 39 | 12 | 8 |
| hospital | 18 | 27 | 36 | 8 | 11 |
| old-age home | 36 | 43 | 9 | 9 | 3 |

|  | occupation | | | | |
|---|---|---|---|---|---|
|  | professional management | technical | skilled | unskilled | never worked |
| community | 10 | 9 | 33 | 14 | 25 |
| hospital | 12 | 23 | 28 | 20 | 17 |
| old-age home | 9 | 17 | 17 | 33 | 24 |

## Medical Care

Generally, the elderly are very set in their ways, and one thing they are extremely particular about is their medical care. Patients, some of whom have had the same physician for over twenty years, are often obligated to see the "house physician" when they move into one of these homes. This is just one example of the difficulties involved in providing optimal health care to the elderly in what really is not a medical institution.

This brings us to the next question: are the health services provided in these homes satisfactory or merely tolerable? According to Townsend in *The Last Refuge*, "health care provisions for residents in old peoples' homes were generally inadequate and often inferior to the level of service provided in the community."[5] When patients are permitted to see their own doctor, the staff is often faced with great confusion, since no two physicians practice medicine the same way. This could account for instances of delay, confusion over drug prescriptions, and much more. But to deny the patient the right to see his or her own physician leads to institutionalism, and that is what group homes try to avoid. The primary consideration should be the patient's care, not the staff's convenience.

According to a recent study of nursing homes, many patients are prescribed hypnotic drugs. Of a total of 1,154 residents in twenty-four homes, 33.5 percent were receiving hypnotic drugs.[6] Do these patients really need such drugs? What accounted for the wide difference in drug prescription practices? Interestingly enough, there was no relationship between the number of general practitioners attending certain homes and the variety of drugs supplied. There was, however, a somewhat paradoxical relationship between the hypnotic usage and the resident's level of dependence. "As a group, the least dependent residents (that is, those with the least degree of mental or physical impairment) showed the highest probability of receiving hypnotics, and the probability of receiving hypnotics was appreciably less in high dependency groups."[7] It is plausible that the prescribing of these drugs is mediated by what the staff feels is necessary.

According to M. G. Clarke, one of the major problems with care for the elderly is overmedication or polypharmacy. Some reasons for anxiety in the elderly, and the prescribing of drugs, are sharing a room with someone they have known only a short while; unfamiliar surroundings; deviating from established daily routines; and sleeplessness. What about drug-induced mental disorder? Thirty-six percent of residents were taking psychotropic medication. The prescribed medication was recorded, but the nonprescribed medication was not. What about the adverse drug reactions that are likely to occur when taking four or more drugs? Shouldn't the staff be aware of overmedication problems and try to reduce the amount of medicine taken? Perhaps prescribing these drugs is intended more for the convenience of the staff than for the patient's primary needs. Are the doctors and other qualified personnel treating a symptom?

The medical treatment of a patient does not stop with physical ailments; the psychological and social effects of being in group homes are tremendous and need to be treated in a similar manner, with follow-up care.

## Placement in Group Homes

### *Psychological Factors*
A survey of one hundred admissions to group homes in Cape Town, South Africa, showed that an "interplay of social, physical, and psychiatric factors was responsible for most of the referrals, although psychiatric factors contributed to more than fifty percent of them."[8] Generally, referrals to these group homes is done by the family physician, a social worker, or another family member. Usually there is a psychiatric team that completes a thorough investigation of the patient to see the extent to which the patient needs to be cared for and the way he or she currently functions in society. Table 3 illustrates the various reasons for referrals by the three groups who make the decision.

**TABLE 3**
**Reasons for Referral[9]**

| | by residents | by informants | psychiatrist assessment |
|---|---|---|---|
| physical condition | 8 | 6 | 6 |
| psychiatric state | 1 | 4 | 4 |
| social circumstances | 19 | 15 | 13 |
| physical condition and social circumstances | 31 | 26 | 25 |
| physical condition and psychiatric state | 0 | 3 | 4 |
| psychiatric state and social circumstances | 4 | 8 | 9 |
| physical condition, psychiatric state and social circumstances | 10 | 38 | 39 |

Statistically, psychiatric problems are not shown to be the primary reason for referrals; however, they are the most commonly used referral. Let us look more closely at such psychiatric problems as dementia. The percentage of patients with dementia varies from 37 to 50.6 in group homes that have moderate to severe cases. This is much higher than the 22 percent of hospital patients and only 5 percent of community respondents.[10] It is clearly a major reason for needing external health care. These patients, interestingly enough, take less psychotropic drugs, but still need round-the-clock care by experienced medical staff. Most of them are in good physical condition, but cannot take care of themselves because of irreversible deterioration of intellectual faculties with concomitant emotional disturbance.

But how do these people like being in a group home compared to nursing homes or living at home? Since dementia is a mental disorder, surveys cannot be judged with great accuracy, but these patients obviously are not getting the social reinforcement they so need. The medical staff merely maintains moderately or mildly demented patients, rather than rehabilitating them. This does not seem fair to patients, for they should have the same rehabilitation opportunity as the physically disabled elderly. Dementia patients show a greater risk of death. Could this be because they undergo no rehabilitation? Most likely it is because they are socially isolated and have no use for communication skills. Dementia, however, has been associated with declining physical ability, which could cause the increased death rate. The number of mentally insecure and disturbed patients is rising, which in turn increases the number of residents of old-age homes with dementia.

Another reason a patient may be in a group home is depression. The Hamilton Rating Scale showed that 25 percent of admissions had moderate to severe symptoms of depression and 14 percent showed mild symptoms.[11] It is important to note that there is no relationship between sex, age, or physical ability in these figures. But those persons showing clinical signs of depression had the same Mental Status Questionnaire scores as patients with dementia. This type of testing can lead to misplacement and incorrect treatment. Luckily, there is a simple cognitive impairment test that can distinguish between the two conditions.

One study found that five residents of a particular home were depressed when they were interviewed. (Depressed in this case means withdrawn or possibly suicidal.) One had no treatment; three were overmedicated and became happier and more lucid; and one refused treatment.[12] Is this really satisfactory medical treatment? There are underlying reasons for these patients to be depressed, and they certainly should not be ignored. Also, these were five residents of one home. The staff should separate these people. Furthermore, couldn't their depression be the reason they are in a group home to begin with? Why should an elderly person infringe on the family's happiness because he or she is depressed? Conversely, perhaps this person is depressed because he or she has been taken from home and familiar surroundings. What is there to be happy about?

Why is it beneficial for the patient to be in a group home rather than some type of an institution, or at home? Granted, living in a group home takes a person away from familiar surroundings, but why can't the patient make the most of the opportunity? It is probably the first time in years this patient can actually socialize with people of the same generation, who know the same songs, movies, athletes, etc. Generally, the older person is alone and really cannot communicate with people two and three generations younger.

The staff working with these people should be older, rather than young people to whom this is just a job. Sure, these homes need qualified personnel, but what better doctors and nurses could there be than those who need to come out of retirement because they themselves are getting depressed? Can institutions provide this type of care? No. They provide physical care and then let the patients sit around and talk each other into even greater depression. What about the depressed patients who are physically able to perform a job? The only thing patients have to do in nursing homes is feed themselves. In a group home situation, there is always a job to do: yard work, cleaning, cooking—jobs that get people's minds off their age. Likewise, there are many jobs to do at home, but often sons and daughters treat their parents as children, which only sinks the patient into deeper depression. The elderly feel completely useless because the people they taught basic chores now feel their parents are too old to competently accomplish the same tasks. But anything is better than being idle. This is all related to Sara Simpson's notion that: (1) the residents' level of depression will be inversely related to their level of engagement, and (2) the residents' level of depression will be inversely related to their engagment in those activities they most enjoy.[13]

The subjects of Simpson's test were from different parts of Newcastle, England, and resided in a home with thirty-eight residents. Their daily activities took place in a large lounge and consisted mostly of free time. The landmarks of the day included three meals, morning coffee, and afternoon tea. There were practically no organized activities. Of the original thirty-eight residents, only thirteen participated in this depression study because of mental impairment or lack of cooperation. Basically, what they were measuring were the different types of social, recreational, and daily living engagements. These included a specific activity, walking with an aid, or just plain smoking. Generally, the depressed resident only had one preferred activity; however, there was a noticeable difference in the preferred activity and the level of the depressed person. Some of the more severely depressed people felt they had no control over their environment, and the nondepressed patients concentrated on self-generated activity and internal ideas such as thinking about things, smoking, or reading.

Simpson found that there was a correlation between the level of depression and the activities the patients enjoyed.[14] Obviously, the same activity will not decrease depression levels for everyone, but having activities in these homes is necessary and beneficial. This example shows how institutions do not focus on positive reinforcement activities, but consider room and board adequate care of the elderly. "The engagement concept has become a popular one. However, care must be exercised lest it becomes yet another convenience label, the use of which might too easily be substituted for proper examination of the concept itself."[15]

*Physical Factors*

We have looked at the psychological reasons people live in group homes, but there are many other reasons as well. Let us examine the physical illnesses that require care. They are usually measured by how much their impairment or incapacity interferes with daily life. Table 4 illustrates the most significant handicaps. The survey compares a similar population (the same age category) living in old-age homes as living in the community.

**TABLE 4**
**Moderate or Severe Physical Incapacity**[16]

|  | *old-age homes percentage* | *community percentage* |
|---|---|---|
| pain | 20 | 18 |
| visual defect | 23 | 10 |
| hearing inpairment | 33 | 9 |
| stiffness/weakness | 57 | 13 |
| dyspnoea | 13 | 11 |
| incontinence | 23 | 0 |

Physical inability is one of the primary reasons for confinement to an old-age home (72 percent). The most common physical ailments include visual and hearing impairments and stiffness and weakness. Other age-related conditions include atherosclerosis, cardiac disease, malignancies, and muscular dysfunction. These unfortunate debilitations are, for the most part, irreversible conditions. Upon entering the home, full examinations are completed to see the extent of their incapacity. (The type of illness has usually already been determined. Interference with day-to-day living generally precipitates entrance to a home.)

Generally, such illnesses predispose the patient to a level of dependency. Studies show that the more useless a patient is made to feel, the more useless he or she becomes. And why shouldn't they become dependent when they are offered little or no rehabilitation training? In institutions such as nursing homes, you do not see Nautilus equipment available for the eighty-year-old quadriplegic. But why should you? He's eighty and his mind is probably gone anyway, right? Wrong. (Although this seems to be the attitude of many Americans.) A brilliant mind might be trapped inside a crippled body, but since we like to stereotype the entire elderly population, we prefer to think that all elderly people have regressed.

If that same eighty-year-old quadriplegic were in a group home, perhaps he would have the opportunity to rehabilitate himself, and his level of dependency would decrease. There is nothing more degrading for an elderly man than to be accompanied to the bathroom by a sixteen-year-old "candy-striper."

These people are not only physically dependent, but emotionally as well because of their environment. Maybe their bodies need Nautilus, but their minds need something too. This is where group homes can be extremely advantageous. Elderly people are in a home with several other people in the same situation. They get positive reinforcement from their contemporaries. At home they probably would have been forced to listen to "Don't do that, Grandpa. I'll do it for you." That would probably have done grandpa more harm than good. He may have trained weeks to do a particular movement to "surprise" his family, but with just a few little words his encouragement would be shot. Nor would he have had the opportunity to be independent in a nursing home. But the group home is perfect. The elderly patient sees his peers trying to rehabilitate themselves and competitive spirit makes him try also. In units where peer groups have a fellowship to offer and resources to share, peer norms spark greater incentive.

Obviously, this particular example does not relate to all the various physical incapacities, but each one has a similar application. What about visually impaired persons in a group home? They can learn to read Braille and become more productive. Grandma can learn to read on her own which would be better than having a family member read to her for the next ten years.

These are just a few ideas on how group homes can be more beneficial than institutions or living at home with physical disabilities.

### Societal Factors

Society plays a major role in a person's decision to reside in a home for the elderly. Income, for example, generally decreases as one gets older. People sixty-five and older live on Social Security and hope that Medicare or other insurance will cover medical costs. Seventy-six percent of a sample population had an annual income of less than $3,000 and many had to spend 50 percent of that income on rent.[17] Statistically, old-age home residents and hospital patients were in the lowest income bracket. It is financially impossible for many of the elderly to manage on their own, and since some of these homes are subsidized by the government, it is a cheaper way for them to live. For the senior citizen who is used to being the breadwinner of a family to suddenly have to get used to living on a small pension is a difficult adjustment.

If the elderly cannot afford monthly nursing home payments, they obviously cannot manage private, round-the-clock nurses to come to their homes. The only answer is a group home. If you have several patients in the same situation, it is much less costly, especially if a government subsidy helps.

What about social isolation? As stated earlier, most of the group home residents are widowed or divorced — in short, alone. One's family plays a very important role in development all through one's life. Why would, or should, the family "disown" an older family member? Only 38 percent of the residents in one study had occasional visits from family; 28 percent never or hardly ever saw family members, only 18 percent were able to say they had reasonably good personal visits of any sort; the rest were socially isolated. Good social contact does not stop with family's and friends' visits; it also includes frequent use of such community facilities as parks or movie theaters.

Another study compared socially isolated persons in hospitals, in group homes, and in the community. Only 19 percent of those in the community were isolated, compared with 32 percent in the hospital and 58 percent in group homes.[18]

Visits from family members followed an interesting pattern. Why would there be more visits to people who were still married, less to the widowed and least to divorced or single persons? It seems inconsistent with patient needs. Table 5 illustrates the family's involvement with patients in the community, in hospitals, and in old-age homes. Clearly, old-age group homes are at a disadvantage.

### TABLE 5
### Family Involvement[19]
(percentage)

|  | *deeply involved* | *ocassional/loose involvement* | *not involved* |
|---|---|---|---|
| community | 62 | 26 | 12 |
| hospitals | 62 | 20 | 18 |
| old-age homes | 34 | 38 | 28 |

Another area where they fall down is outside support from caring people, other than the family. (See Table 6.)

**TABLE 6**
**Support of Caring Person[20]**
(percentage)

|  | strongly supportive | mildly supportive | non supportive | no caring person |
|---|---|---|---|---|
| community | 72 | 18 | 5 | 5 |
| hospital | 71 | 23 | 3 | 3 |
| old-age homes | 14 | 23 | 29 | 34 |

According to these statistics, there is something drastically wrong with our society. Why is it when people need others the most, we turn our backs on them? Are we afraid of the elderly? Do we not want to admit that we ourselves will be there someday? Are we such a youth-oriented society that we cannot appreciate what the elderly have to offer? And even if they do not have a lot to offer, isn't it our job to make their remaining years quality ones? These are all questions individuals must answer for themselves.

### Environmental Factors

The environment is a major influence on group home care. Interaction with the environment forces one to use one's mind. When older people have to cope with appropriate environmental complexity their mental functioning is enhanced. The greater an individual's range and type of impairment, the more significant the environment becomes. Some impairments, in fact, may not be inherent, but rather based on where one lives. Perhaps the expectations of the public and individuals inhibit the responses of the elderly. In institutional settings there are few attempts to motivate creativity, self-reliance skills, and problem-solving techniques. People in homes deserve the same opportunities and activities as everyone else.

An important determinant here is where the homes are located, whether in an urban or a rural setting. In an urban home, the elderly can easily walk to the grocery store, library, etc., but in a rural setting they are prisoners of the home. In nursing homes patients are not allowed to come and go on their own. Of course, there is no need to, because everything the patients needs is nearby, or so the staff thinks. What follows is an example of a patient being treated like a prisoner.

A healthy seventy-seven-year-old woman entered a nursing home so she could be close to her husband. She was forbidden to leave the nursing home, even to go to the library a block away. In the evening she was confined to her bed, which came equipped with guard rails. Because this woman was too frail to take care of her husband by herself and could not afford home care, she and her husband were treated like teenagers.

Few institutions have programs that give the elderly the opportunity to release tension in socially accepted ways, such as family debates, exercise, etc. As a last resort, these patients pace, wander, and even throw food, which is interpreted by officials to mean they are not ready to be in society. Even the chairs they have in institutions arouse undesirable behavior; they are oversized and promote the sedentary behavior we so deplore. In their own homes, they are able to purchase the type of furniture most comfortable to them and in an old-age home they are definitely not consulted in the furnishing of the home.

Society still has not developed the therapeutic potential of the environment. Rather, institutions paint buildings with bright colors and believe this has a psychological effect on the patient. (Psychological studies have shown that the color of a room has an effect on subjects' behavior, but this has an adverse effect when institutions are decorated to look like grade school classrooms at holiday time. All the time, energy, and money have only made it look even more like an institution.) More important is that the patient is made to feel as if in familiar surroundings. Planners and designers need to utilize the potential of the environment. This would cost the institution more money, but the advantage would far outweigh the costs. And it would help alter the public's attitudes on old age. We need to start with the preschoolers and show them growing old does not always mean dementia, disability, deafness or blindness. The public might encourage new expectations of institutions if the media were able to show the public such changes as rehabilitation effectiveness, occupational therapy, speech therapy, dental care, memory development — the list is endless.

More plans for the future could include different organization of furniture. Lounges in institutions are arrranged so cleaning equipment can be easily maneuvered. Anyone who has ever lived in a house knows the time and work involved in cleaning and housekeeping. But that same person knows the self-satisfaction that comes with sharing one's home for dinner or tea. This is another drawback of institutions. The staff is an important part of institutions and should have a role to play in the building's physical design. These people are also role models for the patients, whether they acknowledge it or not, and if they do not take pride in the nursing home, why should the patients?

In conclusion, group homes play an essential role—physiologically, socially, and psychologically—in supplying the health needs of the elderly. These homes serve as an alternative to the impersonal, medically oriented institution, they are the last vestige of the small family group. With all of today's medical technology we must not forget to allow the elderly their human dignity.

# 14

# HOME CARE FOR
# DYING CHILDREN

One dying six-year-old boy asked his mother, "Will it be long now?" She replied, "No, it won't be long." And she carried him into her bed, where he lay between his mother and his father. When the parents awoke a couple hours later, their son had died — peacefully.[1]

O ver two thousand children die from cancer each year in the United States. At the present time, there is no known medical treatment that can reverse the course of cancer in its final stage.[2] Cancer is hard enough for a family to deal with when the patient is an adult; but when the patient is a child, the grief is that much greater.

## Alternative to Hospitalization

Ten years ago, there was no choice as to where a child with cancer would die. A hospital was the only place. Now, however, it is a common practice to bring the child home for his last days of life. According to Ida Martinson, home care can have both psychological benefits in terms of reduced feelings of helplessness for parents, relief of stress for both parents and child, and financial benefits in terms of reduced cost.[3]

Home care helps parents reduce their feelings of helplessness by letting them be the primary caregivers. Parents then feel as if they are doing something to make their child feel comfortable and loved.

When a child is dying in the hospital, doctors tend to stop coming by, nurses turn cold, and the child begins to slip into the pitfalls of hospital bureaucracy. The child is not a patient, just a bed number with a dollar sign over it.

## Effects of Hospitalization on Children and Patients

Several studies have been conducted on the effect of hospitalization on children. It has been stated that a child's greatest fear while in the hospital is that of separation from the mother. The second greatest fear is separation from things associated with the mother — other members of the family, home, and friends.[4] This is where the relief of stress for both the parents and child enters. Children being looked after at the hospital tend to depend on the staff for care and relief from pain. Often, because of this, they then reject their parents, who apparently do not care for them or cannot rid them of their pain and anguish. But when children are looked after in the home, they are in familiar surroundings with familiar people. This sometimes diminishes the pain and makes the child happier. When the child is happy, the parents are happy.

Home care is not easy. It is a very trying time for parents. They are always feeling guilty and asking, "Why us? Why our little boy?" No one can answer these questions. Emily Kulenkamp, while she was recalling what it took to care for her son Eric at home, wrote:

> "This was by far the most difficult task of our lives — but also one of the most important. For us it also fulfilled a need. We were able to give Eric what he wanted — there had been so little we, or anyone else, could do for him — at least we could do that."[5]

## The Nurse's Role in Home Care

The nurse plays a very important role in the ongoing process of home care. She is the main link between the family and the physician in securing medication for the patient. This is important, because pain control is crucial in making home care a success. During the nurse's visits, she instructs the parents on the ways of caring for the child and teaches them how to perform any special techniques, such as administering oxygen. The nurse also performs services the parents cannot.

Although the parent is the principal provider of care for the child, the nurse is on call twenty-four hours a day, seven days a week. He or she comes over to the home whenever the family requests, whatever the reason.

Families receive a tremendous amount of emotional support from the nurse, she who reassures the parents and helps them deal with the death.

When death does occur, the nurse notifies the doctor and takes care of the necessary arrangements, such as informing the mortician. Contact with the nurse does not cease after the child's death. The nurse usually attends the funeral and continues to provide emotional support to the family.

## Benefits of Home Care

From the inception of modern medical care, hospitals have been the setting for the treatment of children with cancer, including those who are terminally ill. The benefit of any continued hospital care is increasingly questioned once it is understood that there is no chance of the cancer being controlled. The trend today is toward alternative care: in the case of the terminally ill child, home care. More and more advantages are being found in relation to the quality of care the child receives and the psychological benefits for the family.

In the recent past, hospitals have been the appropriate place for the ill to become cured and the terminally ill to die. There is no question that the hospital is where the best possible medical treatment can be received. No other institution has the power to prolong life or resuscitate the dying. People, however, increasingly are rejecting hospital care in favor of being allowed to die with dignity and in comfort. Probably one of the most ignored segments of the terminally ill population, in terms of this desire fulfilled, is the youth of our society.

The hospital, though known for its power to care for the sick, has never been strong on giving the psychological support the patient needs. In the case of the dying child, the hospital seems to promote anxiety and discourage its relief. Terminally ill children react more strongly than would be expected to changes in their environment or family, such as fighting between the parents, changes in schools, moving, or separation. The hospital, then, would seem the last place to put the dying child for comfort and prolonged care. The most affected children, emotionally, are those of grade-school age who do not believe the hospital is for their own well-being. They feel they are being punished for the prospect of their own death; their parents are sending them away to die.

Once hospitalized, the pressures of separation and loneliness continue to mount for children. They may be subjected to either partial or total isolation, making it even more difficult for them to adapt to their situation. This feeling is further reinforced when, in the hospital, continuous care by one doctor and regular visits rarely occur. Instead, care is provided by several physicians and there is no continuity. Children then have no one they can identify as their physician, and the patient-physician relationship, which can be so important, is never established.

Home care for the dying child avoids much of the emotional stress of the hospital. This was especially evident when, in a recent study, children dying of cancer who were old enough to express an opinion, all preferred being at home to being in the hospital. At home, children receive a variety of both psychological and social benefits. They are in a family environment where activities that have always been a part of their lives take place. The attention and discipline they are accustomed to is not withdrawn, as in the hospital, which can lead to confusion and unhappiness. At home, children receive the needed security and love that are intrinsic to the home environment.

In the hospital, the affection that children need is often not provided. Terminally ill children want more affection. However, they do not always make this need known. Often, instead of perceiving this greater need for affection, mothers perceive quite the opposite. When this need goes unnoticed, children are lonely and frustrated. This is less likely to occur in the home. There is no nurse who must see to the needs of a number of other patients, no doctor who has other appointments to keep. At home, families can share the responsibilities in the care of dying children, as well as provide love and affection. So, just as the home is the natural place for children to be while living, it can also be a natural one for dying. Hence, children have their parents, they are in an environment of family surroundings, they can eat food they are used to, they are able to pursue normal activities as much as possible, and they can have the company of their brothers and sisters.

## The Family's Reintegration into Society

After the awaited death of the child, the parents and remaining siblings must face the reality that the child is gone forever. They must be reintegrated into the world they left before the child became ill. This is extremely difficult for everyone involved. Ida Martinson, in her book *Home Care for the Dying Child,* said that it is a little easier for the families who chose home care, as opposed to hospitalization, since they were with the child on a twenty-four-hour basis, they saw progress or deterioration that occurred, they knew what to expect and when to expect it.

It is extremely important to tell the remaining siblings, if they are old enough, about the death of their brother or sister, and not just to ship them off to a relative's house in a faraway place. In the long run, the child will cope better with the death and appreciate the honesty and closeness the family will experience.

## The Child's Comfort and the Gratifying of Wishes

One of the primary concerns for parents who are treating their child at home, is for the child to be as comfortable as possible at all times. This comfort includes the gratifying of the child's wishes. For instance, even though the bedroom is the logical place for children to be taken care of, most of the time they prefer to be in the center of family activities. Most patients in home care studies spent their sleeping and waking hours, and eventually died, in the living room or family room.[7] This is one little thing parents can do for their child.

The parents can also try to understand their child. In some cases this may mean understand verbally. Some cancer patients' voices deteriorate so badly that only the mother understands what a child is trying to say. For instance, one little boy's mother knew that her son wanted to read a specific book, but didn't know which one. She brought him several books at a time, until she found the right one.[8]

Little things like this will make the child much happier and, one hopes, a little more comfortable during the last days.

## The Home as a Better Place to Be

Some last considerations to be taken into account are, first, that hospitals are far from the best place for a child to die. According to the study by Ida Martinson et al., parents reported that the hospital was inconvenient expecially when it was far away from the home. This was found to cause stress in the family, because usually the mother would live near the hospital to care for the ill child, while the father was at home caring for the other children. The father would not always understand what the mother was going through, and tended to stray from the care of the ill child. Also, most of the time younger siblings are not allowed in the hospital to visit. If, however, the dying child is cared for at home, there is the parental choice of allowing siblings to be present at the time of death. Most of the time, however, siblings are at school or sleeping when death occurs.[9]

Home care is clearly the best means of care for the dying child. There are many psychological benefits involved with the child dying at home. The parents' feelings of helplessness are greatly reduced. Home care allows parents to feel as if they are doing something to help their child.

The child's greatest fear is a separation from the parents — the sick child is going through a different period and needs the parents' comfort and reassurance. Often, a child who is cared for at the hospital will reject the parents because they are not there to rely upon. The unfamiliar surroundings of the hospital can cause the child to be uncomfortable and scared.

The child who is placed in his home needs an experienced person to help with specialized medical needs. A nurse, who is on call twenty-four hours a day, can provide the family and child not only with medical expertise, but also with emotional support. The nurse can help the family and dying child to deal with death. After the death, nurses make important arrangements, such as informing the physician and mortician of the death. The nurse continues to provide emotional support even after the child's death.

Not only is home care better for the family and child emotionally, it is also more cost-efficient. Whereas insurance usually covers most hospital expenses, only portions of home care are covered. There are considerably fewer costs involved when the child dies at home.

Home care also helps siblings cope with the child's death. When the sick child dies at home, siblings are aware of the situation and are thus able to deal with the death. Visiting children are often not allowed in a hospital. If they are not able to see their brother's or sister's deterioration, death can come as a shock.

A sick child doesn't want to be shut away from the family, but rather wants to be as much a part of the family as before the illness. Parents can help the child by devoting more time to his or her needs and desires.

Finally, the death of one's child is a very personal matter, and for the most part, hospitals are impersonal places that, even at their best, cannot compete with one's own home as a setting both for comfort and privacy.[10]

# 15

# INDEPENDENT LIVING FOR
# THE PHYSICALLY DISABLED

T he sight of a person in a wheelchair shopping for groceries no longer surprises us. We have become accustomed to designated parking places and license plates for the disabled. Ramps for wheelchairs and accessible bathrooms on college campuses are becoming commonplace, and we are no longer shocked to see students with physical disabilities pursuing higher education. These sights, and the rights they represent, are taken for granted by the majority of the population, but they are new, hard-won gains for people with disabilities. Legislation guaranteeing civil rights for disabled people, and the independent living movement itself, are scarcely a decade old.

The independent living movement owes part of its birth and vitality to the civil rights movement. We have seen an expansion of social consciousness with increased civil rights for all citizens during this time, including those with severe physical limitations. Disabled veterans helped to prepare the way for the independent living movement. Severely disabled veterans returned from World War II with pensions and the possibility of an education under the GI Bill. They returned to a society prepared to be sympathetic (especially if the disability was the result of active service), but unprepared to accommodate their disabilities. Few colleges were prepared to accept them, and fewer still were willing to make the necessary physical changes. In the 1940s, disabled veterans and nondisabled protesters in Illinois camped on the lawn of the governor's mansion to gather public support for their desire for an education.[1] The University of Illinois did accept a few disabled students, and those students paved the way for others. Dis-

This chapter was written by Leah Loveday.

*150*

abled veterans have continued to focus society's attention and support for disability issues, and in securing rights for themselves have helped their disabled civilian brothers. Disabled Vietnam veterans have also contributed to the independent living movement, and at some centers have been among the founders.

The first center, and the independent living movement, had its birth in Berkeley, California. During the late 1960s and early 1970s a number of severely disabled young students at Berkeley met at their residence, the local hospital, to discuss their needs. There were no accessible dormitories on campus, and all of these students required attendant care for some of their personal needs. Institutional living was the only option open to them. As they approached their senior year, they began to discuss the possibilities after graduation. Public transportation was not accessible to them. Most public buildings could not accommodate their needs. Without curb cuts, accessible buildings, and transportation, community life was beyond their reach. Employers were reluctant to hire them and unwilling to modify work areas. These young students recognized their needs for housing and attendant care. What were they to do? Their only choice seemed to lie in taking their degrees and returning to life in an institution. They chose instead to become their own advocates and opened the first independent living center. Polling places were inaccessible and these activists could not go to city hall to meet with council members like their able-bodied counterparts in other civil rights movements. Community attitudes began to change; architectural barriers began to give way. Attitudinal barriers also softened as the new independent living center influenced employers and the community. Disabled people in other parts of the country began to flock to them. Some stayed in the new atmosphere of freedom, while others returned home with the seeds for new centers. Experimental centers began in Houston, Texas, and in Boston, Massachusetts.

The philosophical concepts and the practical implications of the independent living center are unique, even radical, among organizations formed to meet the needs of the severely physically disabled. The center at Berkeley was organized by a group, with everyone contributing—a group of *disabled* people. The organizers, and most of the eventual staff and board members, were disabled people who advocated for their own needs. Most organizations formed to serve people with disabilities are founded and staffed by able-bodied people.

Funds for these organizations are raised by capitalizing upon the disabilities and appealing to the sentiments, emotions, and consciences of the nondisabled. Disabled people are not expected to take part in the fund raising, other than as models for posters, and are passive recipients of the generosity of others. Independent living focuses upon ability and employability and asks that all involved — whether staff, clients, board members, or fund raisers — see and accept each other as peers. Disabled people, and able-bodied supporters, both take responsibility for every aspect of an independent living center, including fund raising. New sources of funding had to be developed, as an independent living center could not depend upon the mass appeal of a sentimental campaign.

Most independent living centers began through federal grants established through the 1978 amendments to the 1973 Rehabilitation Act. Several important pieces of legislation have been signed into law during the last decade, largely due to the efforts of disabled activists. Civil rights for people with disabilities were omitted from the 1964 Civil Rights Act, but nearly ten years later, the 1973 Rehabilitation Act extended civil rights to prohibit discrimination in education, employment, and transportation for disabled citizens. Nearly four years passed before the regulations of this important act were signed into effect, and disabled activists dramatized their requests with some of the same methods used by other civil rights movements before them. Sit-ins were held in Washington to protest the delay, and though the demonstration did not meet with the violence of other civil rights movements, the participants suffered considerable hardship as promised food and drink was either withheld or intercepted by the police, while demonstrators were not allowed to leave, or food vendors to enter.[2] The regulations were eventually signed into law. As amended in 1978, the act affects services funded by grants to states (Title VII), affirmative action (Section 503), and nondiscrimination (Section 504a. Section 504 particularly prohibits discrimination on the basis of a person's disability in any program receiving federal assistance. This legislation is so important that, whenever possible, independent living centers and transitional living centers offer training and information on Section 504.

Under Section 504, mass public transportation must be made accessible to people with disabilities, whereas local governments are allowed a good deal of flexibility in complying with this. This policy is still controversial, with many areas fearing the expense of modified vehicles, and is a source of frustration to disabled people and a cause of much litigation. When the expense of modification is seen in broader terms, the amount seems quite small, for it is far less expensive to society for a disabled person to live independently than in a state-supported institution (as noted by the United States Commission on Civil Rights). Disabled people cannot maintain employment, and become taxpayers, without transportation. Unfortunately, accessible transportation is still a dream in many areas.

Another major hurdle to full community integration has been architectural barriers. The Architectural Barriers Act of 1968, as amended, requires that all buildings funded by the federal government be accessible to disabled people, and usable by them, in accordance with government standards. The 1973 Architectural and Transportation Compliance Board was empowered in 1978 to establish guidelines and requirements for accessible design. This legislation has also been controversial, and noncompliance with it continues to be an obstacle for physically handicapped people. Sometimes professionals are aware of this law, but either do not see its necessity or are ignorant in its application. For example, a southwestern university constructed a new student union after enactment of these regulations. As the university received federal funds, the building was designed with accessible bathrooms and widened doorways to accommodate wheelchairs. Unfortunately, it was also designed with planters in front of all doorways so that those in wheelchairs could not enter. Sit-ins were held by disabled students and able-bodied supporters, and the planters were removed from the new building. Architectural barriers and too few sidewalk curb cuts continue to limit the activities and opportunities of disabled people.

Employment and educational opportunities have been slowly opening up for disabled Americans since the passage of the 1975 Education for All Handicapped Children Act and Section 504 for adults. Visible barriers such as buildings and sidewalks are slow to change, and subtle barriers of prejudice and stereotype, are often slower. Equal opportunity has been mandated only for programs receiving federal support, and sometimes there is discrimination in these areas as well. For example, one highly capable woman was released from her job at the United States Post Office after the onset of her disability. After twelve years there she was entitled to a pension, which she received.

Her condition is now medically stable, yet after much negotiation she has not been rehired. Her twelve years had led to a highly responsible position, yet the only offers from the Post Office have been menial positions, or a responsible position at much lower pay. She is very knowledgeable about Section 504 and continues to negotiate for her former position (or a comparable position), which would be unaffected by her disability. She uses a crutch now and cannot stand for long periods of time, but her energy and capacity for work are unlimited and very little accommodation is required. Such disappointments are common, even worse when the former job was in private industry and there is no hope of rehiring, or when the disabled person cannot find employment. Unemployment and underemployment is disproportionately high for people with disabilities, who frequently earn less than their able-bodied counterparts with the same skills and education. [3]

Unfortunately, poverty often accompanies disability, as do myriad other difficulties. Assistance programs do not discriminate against the disabled person, but the program may be housed in physical surroundings or involve an application procedure difficult for some disabled people. Some programs, such as Social Security Insurance and Social Security Disability Insurance, contain work disincentives, so that the disabled worker limited to part-time hours may be penalized or lose assistance altogether. If unable to perform full-time work, the disabled person either lives on a low income with assistance, or on a low income with part-time wages.

Physically disabled persons face other challenges to independent living. Some grew up in an era of custodial care for disability, or a restrictive and protective environment, and may have difficulty adjusting to a self-directed life. Others are faced with sudden, traumatic disabilities, as medical technology is more able to save victims of accidents or survivors of formerly fatal diseases. There are problems of adjustment, problems of interaction with the rest of society, physical and emotional hurdles to a full and independent life. Some severely disabled people may need the care of an attendant in order to live independently.

Independent living centers deal with all of these problems with a wide range of programs and supportive services and more, because most centers employ a qualified staff of people with a variety of disabilities. Staff and clients are peers. Staff members know which parts of the city are accessible, how it feels to receive financial assistance, about living on a low income, the nuances of the city's transportation system, the physical and emotional difficulties their peers face. Staff members also serve as role models for disabled people living a self-directed life. It is important that the director of the agency have a disability or else have personal experience with disability. It is a delight for a disabled person to enter a center for the first time and perhaps see that the director has the same disability, or that the counselor/advocate knows about disability from firsthand experience, or that the coordinator of the attendant referral program also requires an attendant, and to see people with many kinds of disabilities busy with projects or socializing comfortably. Also, firsthand experience with disability puts the staff in touch with a network of community resources not listed in textbooks. The new client quickly feels accepted and at home.

Ideally, the board of an independent living center is comprised of disabled and able-bodied members. Disabled people should be recruited as board members whenever possible.

Before describing the programs available at a typical independent living center, it is interesting to take a look at the grass-roots beginnings of many centers. Some report beginning services in an old warehouse, or in a small office in a low-rent area. Like the hospice movement in this country, the independent living movement has seen a number of centers open all across the nation, organized by small groups of concerned citizens. Unlike the hospice movement, the independent living movement is organized by the very people they are intended to serve.

A center in the Southwest was organized by two men and a woman in wheelchairs, one a disabled Vietnam veteran. All three contributed their time and money to start the center in one of the poorest areas of town. The tiny center could not afford heat in the winter or air conditioning in the summer, which is a hardship in the Southwest. Volunteers were the only staff, and at first the center was not recognized by the community. They were not included in meetings of agencies serving disabled people and were not given referrals. The community saw them as a small group of loud, disabled people. At first they were only able to provide a hot line of information and referral, and the hotline itself gathered information on the needs of disabled people. The center saw which needs were not being met by existing agencies and other gaps in care in the community. Other disabled volunteer staff members gathered, and soon one woman began to organize specific individual areas of service as staff developed expertise. She visited a large number of community agencies in order to further research community needs and to insure that the independent living center did not duplicate services.

She learned how to write grants, and nine months after its beginning in a small town office, the new center had Title VII funds. With funds from other grants as well, the center was able to move to a more accessible location and could begin hiring staff in a variety of areas. In less than four years the center has grown, and though not luxurious, now has offices and a professional staff of disabled people providing counseling, advocacy, paralegal aid, instruction in living skills, job placement, recreation programs, housing and attendant referral, as well as wheelchair repair and a service that provides home modifications to low-income disabled city residents. Over 90 percent of the staff have disabilities, most have college degrees, and some have advanced degrees. Many work part time to accommodate the center's small budget, as well as their own disabilities. People with a wide range of disabilities are served and no one is turned away. All services except wheelchair repair are free to clients.

Part of the basic philosophy of independent living is self-direction by the disabled person. Clients are not passive "patients"; they actively determine their own goals and priorities. They participate in planning and determining their individual working plan at the center, and in many centers a contract is made between the staff person and the client. This contract, or work plan, is reviewed and revised periodically. Though centers may offer different programs, each reflects the goal of independence for the disabled person. Many centers offer training designed to increase independence, such as budgeting, nutrition, menu planning, shopping and cooking, driver's education or bus training, and the legal rights of a disabled person. Individuals are encouraged to ask questions, to be assertive, and to get the information they need. Some learn to find out more about the medications they receive and treatments open to them. Those who need to further their social skills may participate in the social/recreational program. Some centers offer training for volunteers, which is a good way to develop job readiness. Most centers provide peer counseling and support groups to share the problems and concerns of disability.

Political participation may be encouraged among clients informally, and voter registration may take place at the center. Sometimes people from the center participate in community workshops on civil liberties, or may circulate a petition for requests such as accessible city transportation.

There are numerous programs found in some centers, though not in all. Employment services are sometimes available, as are consultants or programs for modification of work or home areas. Some centers offer therapy, such as speech or occupational therapy.

Independent living centers are helping to change society's image of the disabled person, and through their programs are changing the self-image disabled people have of themselves. All are seen as having the right and the freedom to achieve to their maximum potential. Full participation in the community and the freedom to choose individual lifestyles are not only achievable, but practiced by staff members and clients with disabilities. Independent living centers demonstrate that the old practice of segregated institutional life for people with disabilities is obsolete.

Perhaps the key program at the majority of independent living centers, and the program that makes independent living a reality for many, is attendant referral. A personal-care attendant provides services for elderly and physically disabled adults, which may include bathing, dressing, transfer, toilet assistance, grooming, and perhaps feeding, shopping, or meal preparation. "Attendant care is viewed as an alternative to institutionalization."[4] Many people with physical disabilities have been institutionalized when attendant care was not available. Institutionalization is needlessly expensive for the state and needlessly confining for the disabled person. Severely disabled people are usually medically stable and do not need medical supervision, but they do need assistance because of physical limitations. They are not sick, but have physical limitations.

Attendant care itself is not new; aides have been providing service in institutions or in homes under the direction of a medical supervisor for a long time. Attendant referral programs, as developed in many independent living centers, are distinctive because the attendant is under the direction of the disabled consumer. There are many home health agencies that train attendants, but they are supervised and trained by the agency's supervisor, usually a registered nurse. Duties are clearly delineated by the agency. The aide is employed by the agency and is responsible to the staff, not to the disabled person. The person receiving services is a passive patient, with little or no input on the care given. Outside control of attendant care keeps the recipient dependent and may foster a lack of initiative in other areas as well. If a person's whole daily routine is in another's hands, and there are few choices about the time of rising, bathing, eating, or when and how other activities are to take place, there is little room for expression of an individual lifestyle. When the details of daily life are managed by someone else, the disabled person gets little practice in making personal decisions and may have a harder time participating in the community.

The concepts of independent living are just the opposite. Just as independent living centers encourage self-direction in other areas—such as setting goals for counseling, employment, or education—the center encourages disabled consumers to direct their own personal care. Needs vary considerably among disabled people, so needs for attendant services vary also. A young woman with cerebral palsy, for instance, understands her own health needs and has the intelligence and determination to pursue a master's degree. She walks easily and handles her own toilet needs independently, but needs to be fed. She does not want or need a full-time attendant, just assistance for a few brief periods each day. Another might require a few intervals of more time-consuming care a day. For instance, a young man is a medically stable quadriplegic who drives his own adapted van to work at an independent living center. While at work he manages his own needs and functions independently as he directs the attendant referral program. He employs an attendant who helps him to dress and prepare for work in the morning, and to retire in the evening. Because of his schedule and needs, he employs three attendants, one for the morning routine, one for the evening, and another for weekends. A third example is an elderly person severely debilitated by a long illness. She needs an attendant for several hours in the morning, noon, and evening for personal as well as household care, and is thus able to continue to live independently at home.

To accommodate a diversity of consumer needs, common sense would indicate that the program be geared to the individual and not the other way around. Attendant referral programs at independent living centers give the responsibility for hiring, training, and paying the attendant to the disabled consumer. A few independent living centers have contracts to pay attendants, but the disabled person is usually the employer. Centers encourage disabled consumers to be in charge of their own lives and to carefully note their needs in order to train an attendant.

Centers assume that those who understand their own health care and personal needs are the best qualified to train an attendant to perform that care. Therefore, the center trains the disabled consumer to interview potential attendants, to check references, to discuss the care required and such matters as taxes and employee benefits. The center does not hire the attendant, but maintains a list of available people and pertinent information, such as the care the person is willing to perform, hours desired, areas of town available, and wage desired. Some centers interview potential attendants; many leave that duty to the disabled consumer. Members of the attendant referral program make sure that the disabled consumer understands the hiring procedure and offer guidance and suggestions for training and for keeping an attendant. If a consumer has severe disabilities, someone from the center may visit the person's home, both for training in becoming an employer, in the concepts of independent living, and perhaps to make suggestions for home modifications. Many centers also offer follow-up services, as well as a three-part contract for the consumer, the attendant, and the center.

Attendants at many centers are also offered services and may receive training in various aspects of care. At some centers regularly scheduled sessions deal with such aspects of care as correct lifting methods, methods of transfer, and bowel, bladder, and skin care. Disabled employers fine-tune the training to their own individual needs and preferences. They also determine the hours of care and arrange their own daily schedule. Attendants are accountable to their disabled employers.

One of the basic concepts of the attendant referral program is that disabled people are the employers and they direct and control the service they need. Unfortunately, many third-party payers do not hold the same concept and will pay only if a doctor prescribes nursing care. Care is then in the hands of the medical profession, which may not be necessary. It may also be unnecessarily expensive. Title XX funds may also be used for attendant services in some states, but the direction of these services may be in professional rather than consumer hands. Also, disabled people run the risk of losing attendant care benefits if they accept employment. Attendant-care costs may make it unfeasible for disabled persons to work even if they are otherwise qualified and able. Health care providers of attendant care prefer to keep services under professional, rather than consumer, control. Pressured by such interests, third-party payers, may continue to finance medically controlled attendant care. The independent living movement needs to continue to find community and legislative friends for this vital service.

To be independent, disabled persons need to be responsible for their health and personal care, for their own bodies. Unnecessary medical or agency intervention fosters dependence. Responsibility for personal care is essential to an individual's self-respect and self-esteem.

Attendant care programs contribute directly to the deinstitutionalization of the disabled, to paraphrase the attendant coordinator from a center in Ann Arbor, Michigan. As he says, "With adequate home care, the overwhelming majority of persons with *physical* disabilities can live very successfully outside of institutions." We've seen the wisdom and efficiency in the last decades of community rather than institutional life for people with disabilities. May we soon acquire the wisdom to finance consumer-based services, rather than unnecessary medical care.

Some attendant-referral programs, and many independent living centers, also keep a file of low-cost, accessible housing. A disabled person may have the skills for independent living but nowhere to go in the community if accessible housing is not available. Some need an additional step between a dependent living situation and independence. Transitional rehabilitation programs attempt to provide temporary group-living situations and other services. Disabled individuals who may not be able to move directly into an independent living situation include those who have lived for a long time in an institutional setting, young adults with congenital disabilities who have always been cared for at home, and those who need more time and specialized services.

Philosophically, transitional rehabilitation is nearly the same as the independent living movement and also seems to have a little in common with the hospice movement. Like their peers at independent living centers, disabled residents in a transitional setting are trained to be independent. They are not patients, and they actively determine their goals during their stay at a transitional residence. Client and staff write a contract together, which is reviewed and changed monthly. Programming is flexible and individualized. As in the hospice movement, staff members are seen as part of a multidisciplinary team, including the physician. The concept is wholistic, so that every area of life receives attention.

Residents learn to manage their own health care, to take medication independently. Programs, as in an independent living center, reflect the goal of self-direction and include self-care skills, driver education, vocational guidance, sports, attendant-care training, and community-living classes. Residents develop problem-solving ability and, through these programs, the self-confidence to live independently. Counseling is available, as well as traditional therapies found in other rehabilitation programs.

An article on Courage Residence, in Minnesota, indicates that the typical client is between twenty and twenty-four years of age, has a severe disability, stays at the residence for an average of nine months, and that the majority are able to maintain an independent living situation after discharge. A follow-up study found that 74 percent were living independently a year later.[5]

Transitional residences can be highly successful when there is an accessible community waiting for the residents after discharge. The operating concepts of a transitional residence seem very compatible with the independent living movement. Yet brochures seem to indicate an able-bodied staff with disabled clients, though there are disabled people serving on the governing boards. One hopes that there are at least some staff members with disabilities (and abilities) who can serve as role models for clients with disabilities. Also, it may be difficult for a live-in center, even with high ideals, not to institutionalize to some degree. As most residents stay for less than a year, the danger seems small, and it is to the credit of a transitional residence that it remains truly transitional and contributes to the success of the independent living movement.

There have been enormous successes for the independent living movement and for individuals with disabilities in our recent history. Severely disabled people have moved out of the isolated institutions in vogue for a century and into colleges, private apartments and homes, marriages, and a variety of jobs not thought possible a short time ago. Independent living centers have trained countless individuals who would have been institutionalized otherwise to hire their own atten- dants to direct their own care. People with disabilities have become their own advocates, have changed their civil rights status and the laws affecting them, and have opened community doors long closed to them. They've requested, inspired, and sometimes designed equip- ment that allows them to utilize more of their abilities. Architecture for public buildings and accessible transportation concretely symbol- ize this changed environment.

It would seem that utopia is here. But let's look again. What are some of the problems facing independent living centers and people with physical disabilities? How will other environmental factors af- fect the independent living movement — changes in medical technol- ogy, the economic climate, and the attitudes and mores of the "nor- mal" population? The first question can best be answered by people with disabilities actively involved in the independent living move- ment. The second question will find no firm answer here, but we can look at the present and find hints of the future.

The brick walls of the old institutions are crumbling fast, but full community acceptance is still found more on paper than in practice. The new client's enthusiasm and euphoria during the first visits to an independent living center reflect the novelty of acceptance. "I didn't know places like ths existed!" a middle-aged woman recently exclaimed to a staff member. "I thought it was all over for me after my stroke, that I'd be useless. My kids treat me different now; they are afraid to tell me things. My grandchildren make fun of me because I walk dif- ferent. My boyfriend left. He didn't want someone who couldn't walk fast or dance like I used to." She was amazed to see staff members with more severe disabilities and to find that the director of the center had also survived a stroke. Her reaction and experience are repeated in the lives of many, many people with disabilities.

Aniek, a strikingly pretty Amerasian young woman in her twenties, directs several programs at an independent living center and has seen much discrimination in her own personal life. As employment coun- selors at the center, she and other staff members also see the effects of subtle forms of discrimination. As part of her job, Aniek visits schools and community organizations when a speaker is requested. Little children openly express their astonishment that she is pretty, wears nice dresses, and has long red fingernails — because she uses a wheelchair. She tells them stories of isolation at parties, of young, liberal, educated people moving aside at her approach and ending conversations quickly. She tells them of going from an active social life at a "crip" school to invisibility during her first year of college. The children are surprised that she dates (actually she is much in demand with eligible men, both with and without disabilities). Teenagers are interested to learn that she has sex, and she demolishes the old concept of a person with disabilities as asexual. Her eager young listeners are less likely than their parents to be embarrassed and uncomfortable and cruelly isolating with a disabled person.

Aniek feels that community acceptance is one of the major problems faced by "disabled folk." As she says, "Employers want a super crip, someone gorgeous, brainy, lots of education, and in their twenties. They either hire people with developmental disabilities (retarded), or educated disabled people for minimum wages. We have to work so hard to prove that we can do it. We have to look so perfect. I have to dress like this to show that disabled folks are to be taken seriously as professional."

Professionals, like Aniek, often face uncomfortable or even comical situations because of others' reactions to their disabilities. Many prepare in advance and learn how to make others feel more comfortable. One agency director with a physical disability took her able-bodied secretary with her to a community meeting. At first those at the meeting thought the secretary was the director and spoke only to her. Fortunately, the director has a good sense of humor and uses it to help people recover from their embarrassment.

It would be easy to continue recording similar incidents, as people with even minor physical limitations are greeted with discomfort and aversion. Many people in our culture are unfamiliar with disabled people, particularly if they went to segregated schools or grew up in an area where disabled people lived in institutions or stayed at home. With deinstitutionalization and accessible transportation and buildings, those with physical disabilities are more visible. People with disabilities are seen more frequently in the arts today. A cartoon character might use a wheelchair, or movies might feature someone with a disability (though often "super crip"). There are even toys now with prostheses. The television series "Hill Street Blues" featured a man in a wheelchair and portrayed him realistically, without paternalism or sentiment. Attitudes are changing, but as Aniek says, it may take a long time before there is complete integration. Meanwhile, "disabled folk" continue to face a difficult hurdle to employment and community acceptance.

The trend seems to be toward increased community acceptance. No one hates disabled people, and discomfort and embarrassment can diminish with exposure. The old stereotypes give way as "disabled folk" are seen as people with the same mix of virtue and vice as everyone else, neither heroes nor saints nor degenerate and degraded because of physical impairment.

Transportation also continues to be a major barrier for disabled people. Most disabled people cannot afford an adapted van for those with electric wheelchairs, or an adapted car for those with manual wheelchairs. Many must rely upon city transportation, which may include special buses especially for disabled people, or adapted city buses for the whole population. Professionals in wheelchairs may find it difficult to schedule meetings outside of their offices because of transportation problems. Appointments at independent living centers are often canceled for the same reason. It is often difficult to plan social events for center clients when there is no reliable transportation system. Transportation is indispensable for a disabled person conducting a job search. Volunteer opportunities are limited without transportation. In fact, full community participation is impossible unless adequate transportation is available to every disabled person.

Accessible transportation, as well as employment possibilities, are affected by the economic climate. It is obvious that jobs will be scarce for everyone, and especially for the disabled worker, in a tight economy. Programs and services for the disabled, including transportation, are likely to be restricted during a tight economy, and it seems that many independent living centers will face funding problems within the next few years. The original establishment grants under Title VII will be running out soon, and centers may have to cut back staff and services if other grants and funds do not become available.

There are many humanitarian and practical reasons for continued funding of independent living centers. Centers have contributed directly and indirectly to deinstitutionalization for many people, thereby saving the state a good deal of money. Community living is far less expensive than institutional life. No other community service provides training in hiring an attendant and in self-directed personal care. The state saves again when the disabled consumer chooses attendant care rather than a needlessly expensive medically directed service. Many services are provided at independent living centers for people who do not fit into traditional rehabilitation agencies. Disabled people are more likely to contribute to their communities through the efforts of independent living centers.

Centers vary considerably in the services they provide. Some people who have long been involved in the independent living movement see this as a problem. They feel that services are fragmented and that there are no uniform standards. Others see this diversity as a plus and feel that centers reflect local needs more accurately with flexible programs. They also see unity in diversity, for though centers provide different services in different locations, the same philosophy unites them all. All centers share a belief in the self-direction of the disabled person. It seems likely that a service devoted to independence for people with disabilities will also be independent, and independent centers need the freedom to develop new services as they are needed.

We cannot foresee totally the needs of the future. The disabled population is changing as former crippling diseases such as polio have been nearly eradicated. Medical technology has developed the ability to save people who have been severely injured; but many of these people are left with permanent physical disabilities. For them disability is a sudden trauma. Also, many survive formerly fatal childhood diseases well into adulthood (such as cystic fibrosis, muscular dystrophy, and some forms of cancer). Some physical disabilities turn into other disabilities, as is the case for those who survive cancer but lose part of their bodies. It is likely that the disabled population will continue to change as the cause and treatment of disability changes. Services, such as independent living centers, will have to be flexible to meet future needs.

The present holds the seeds of endless future possibilities. Perhaps medical technology will change the nature of physical disability by making such devices as the bionic hand of *Star Wars* Luke Skywalker available to nonmovie heroes. Perhaps transportation will become accessible when conveyances yet to be invented appear on the market. Perhaps the goals of the original independent living centers will become universally realized, with self-determination and independence a basic fact of a disabled person's life, with complete community acceptance and participation of all citizens, and with full opportunities in employment and education.

# 16

## THE MARKETING
## OF HOME CARE

A merican consumers are faced with many choices today. Large industries and corporations constantly are trying to get consumers to buy their products. How do they sell a product or service? Industries and corporations try to convince consumers that their products and services are better than all the others through the use of such marketing techniques as innovative television commercials, radio jingles and songs, advertisements and coupons offering special discounts—all of which make one product more desirable than another. Because of the wide variety of products available to the consumer, marketing and advertising are essential to the success of selling those products and services. Since marketing is indispensable in the industrial, commercial world, it is logical to assume that it would have a valuable application when selling home health care services to consumers—patients and nonpatients, who have a choice.[1]

Until recently, society has favored institutionalization, and home care has been viewed as an option or alternative to hospital or institutional care. But home care is the normal environment for the patient, and its advocates are trying to convince the consumer that all other facilities are in fact, alternatives to being at home. Just as in industry, however, it is difficult to market a new concept. Industries fear that their products will not be successful, and home health care agencies fear that consumers will not use their services. The only way the population at large will learn about services available to them is through education, advertising, and exposure to the public. It is a vicious cycle, for only when people know what is available to them can they make a decision about what they want.

Hospitals and other institutional facilities, with their medical and technological resources, have been considered the only options for those seeking medical service. Recently, home health care services have been considered an essential part of the health care system. Why? Home health services and other health and social services provide an economical and desirable way of meeting health care needs. Also, the home environment is important in promoting health and it facilitates the healing process. It also allows the family to become involved in the care of the patient, so the patient and family are not isolated from one another. Home health care takes into consideration the whole patient: body, mind, and emotions. All of these are important in treating illness. The development of home health services, aimed at meeting these needs, testifies to the importance of home care. But home care services are not new. Consumers are only now becoming aware of the necessity to develop new patterns of care that meet the patients' needs and are moving toward the notion of home care. Thus, with the development of home care, patients have an option—home or hospital.[2]

Changes in social and cultural patterns, and health and economic reasons, have increased the operation of hospital facilities and the cost of hospital care. One social change, for instance, is that the life expectancy of the population and the number of those suffering from long-term illnesses has increased. Present patterns of care for this population are "institution-centered," "disease-centered," and "procedure-centered." They do not meet the needs of the individual. Many individuals would not require hospitalization if care in the home were available. In addition, their progress may be even better in the home than in the hospital, for in a suitable home environment, many patients make rapid physical and mental improvements. These patients often are not aware of other services available to them. Home health care must be promoted. Increase in long-term illness and the rise in the average life expectancy suggests that services that provide nurses and other home helpers should be organized to reduce the rising hospital costs and emphasize the individualization of treatment. By building a more rational, comprehensive, efficient, and humane system for delivering health services, the consumer would be faced with a range of alternatives, including the hospital, the nursing home, and a system of home health care. Because of current health trends and the future projections of health care needs, home care can and should be viewed as a marketable product.[3]

## Marketing Strategy for Home Care

Marketing is an essential part of management for any agency, including home health agencies. A basic principle of marketing, as in management, is "there is no one best way of doing things." When marketing a product or service, it is important to realize that situations and cases vary. For example, a seventy-eight-year-old woman with arthritis will have different health care needs than an eight-year-old boy with terminal cancer. Those in the field of home care must maintain interest and keep up with the best ways to serve the medical needs of the patient. It is essential to be able to answer the following three questions: Who needs medical attention? What do they need? What is the best way to fulfill those needs? In order to market services and extend them to the community at large, a marketing strategy is necessary. For example, industries marketing a product need to identify the product, who the product is for, and why it is needed. Once this is established, the organization decides how to reach the consumer. Similarly, the home health care product is identified as a service, a service that generally is not purchased until it is needed. It is a product, though, that the consumer/patient must be able to identify and recognize as an available service if the need arises. The next step in marketing is to establish the purpose of the marketing plan. The final step is to develop a marketing plan.[4]

### *Definition of Home Health Care*

Home health care services are those required because an individual is "homebound and requires home health services on a visiting basis to meet his health care needs." Home health care services are suited to meet the comprehensive health care needs of the individual. Programs attempt to supply medical services to patients in their homes in order to shorten the length of the hospital stay, to speed recovery and to offer community health services for those who do not need hospital care but are too ill or unable to visit their physicians. Home care services are usually provided for the purpose of "promoting, maintaining or restoring health or minimizing the effects of illness." Initially, the patient requires a broad array of home health services. Then as the patient begins to recover he or she continues to need services, but the services provided vary with the patient's condition. Home care can be considered a health care service that benefits the entire community.[5]

## The Goal of Home Health Care

The overall goal of home health care is to "insure that the needs of the patient are being met by providing the proper health services." With the increase in diseases that demand long rehabilitation periods, for health and economic reasons there is a great need to see that after-care is as effective as possible. The purpose of the home care program, then, is to coordinate and provide these professional health services to patients in their homes. With this goal in mind, home health care has allowed patients to live and be treated at home with dignity, it has spared them the loneliness of institutional care, and it has allowed them to be as independent as possible. It has also prevented or postponed disability, prevented or shortened institutionalization, maintained the family unit and included the family in treating the illness, and finally, helped patients to economize on medical costs. These are goals that home care programs hope to achieve. By offering these services and demonstrating that they are extremely effective in meeting the needs of the patient's mind, body, and emotions, providers have good reason to promote and sell the concept of health care.[6]

## The Purpose of the Marketing Plan

Now that the product is identified, the next step is to establish the purposes of health agencies' marketing plans. The marketing plan is to deliver home health care. The purposes:

1. Generate revenue. The agency needs to make money in order to pay the employees. Without people, you are without an agency. Thus, an agency with a successful market plan will make a profit.

2. In order to generate a profit it is important to get the services to those who need them. Since home care is generally a service that consumers do not want to pay for, they won't unless they need it.

3. Build an image and credibility. If consumers believe that the program or agency is legitimate, they are more likely to use it, so the agency makes money. "Reputations make or break an agency."

4. The most important purpose of the marketing plan is to meet competition. Home health care agencies must compete with hospitals and other institutional facilities for multibillion-dollar sources of federal money created by Medicare/Medicaid. For the most part, establishing a good plan will let the agency meet the competitor problem.

**5.** Growth indicates success. Home care agencies hope to expand, for this indicates a need for services, which in turn signifies a profit.[7]

It is important that the agency know what it wants to achieve before developing a market plan.

### Identify Need/Future Projection

Once the purposes of the marketing plan have been established, one area to examine is whether there is a demand and a market for the service. Before actually trying to set up a marketing plan and sell a product, the organization must know if the consumers, will need or use the product or service they wish to produce.

Already the need for home health care is limitless. Consumers are looking for alternatives to reduce medical costs and to return to a more humanistic approach to medicine. In addition, home health care represents a choice of services for many patients with a variety of health problems. Home health agencies are on the rise due to the increasing need for and utilization of their services. Since the need for home health care is expanding, agencies should have strategies and long-range plans for their growth. In order to meet the future demands in home health care, agencies should know:

**1.** the life situation of clients. The elderly population is increasing and there has been an increase in terminal illnesses.

**2.** the community's health structure, the economic potential, and the value placed on health. Health care is a service people usually do not purchase unless there is a need for it, so it is important to know if the community places a high value on health and will pay for care needed.

**3.** how professionals and nonprofessionals view the health care agency. Many physicians fear competition with agencies because it will lower their income. In order to be successful in the long run, agencies need to overcome physicians' fears and gain their support.

**4.** how to create a demand for the agency's services and how to compete with institutional care. Since there is already an urgent need for alternatives to institutional care, it is not necessary to induce demand. It is necessary, however, that the consumer be aware of services available to them. Since a future and present need have already been established, the only way in which to sell the service is to market it.[8]

## Identify the Consumer

Once it is established that home health care services are and will be utilized, it is important to know who will be using the services so providers will know at which group(s) of the population to direct their marketing plan. Although there is an urgent need, lack of awareness of the availability of services results in underuse. Therefore, find out who uses the services and make them aware.[9]

## The Elderly

Senior citizens are one natural market for home health care services. Misconceptions tend to discourage home care for the elderly. People often believe that the ills of the elderly are imaginary and they are just trying to get attention. Another myth is that managing the ills of the elderly is too difficult and bothersome, thus the tendency toward institutionalization. Reduced employment and retirement of the elderly has made it difficult for older people to adjust to the social and economic problems of long-term illness, so they wind up in institutions. According to the American Public Health Association, "10–25% of persons in institutions could live at home if appropriate services were available." Organized health care should direct their services toward the elderly and provide a means of meeting the health, social, and economic needs of that segment of our population. With the over-seventy-five population increasing, producers of home care services should plan now to improve the variety and quality of care available.[10]

## The Terminally Ill

The increase in the number of terminal illnesses has also increased the need for delivering services to patients in their homes. With the high cost of institutional care, and for psychological and emotional reasons, many terminally ill patients prefer to be at home with those they love and in surroundings familiar to them. In addition, the family can work out its reaction to grief and the patient can die with dignity. Terminal patients can benefit greatly from these services if they are available to them.[11]

## Children

Another natural market for home care services are children. Home care benefits many groups of people, but children may be the ones who benefit the most. Children have little experience with being away from home and tend to feel secure only with their family and in their home. Children need delicate care, particularly when ill, so being away from loved ones could be very traumatic. Home care provides a familiar setting and allows the family to help the child adjust emotionally.[12]

### The Handicapped

Although handicapped people do not use much institutional care, they are a large group of home health care consumers. Home care has helped disabled patients to resume participation in their jobs, education, and social lives.[13] Thus, home health agencies must not neglect making their services available to the disabled.

## Developing a Marketing Plan

The marketing plan is based on the internal and external data collected through market research when examining whether there is a demand and a market for the product or service. In industry, in order to introduce the consumer to the services available, personal selling by various means of promotion and communication is directed to potential consumers. One area the agency is concerned with is advertising and promotion of the service. Industries rely heavily on advertising through television, radio, and magazines. Home health agencies do not advertise this way, but instead rely more on personal selling through direct communication between the consumer and a salesperson. The job of the salesperson is to "act as a catalyst" and bring the services to the consumer. The hospital coordinator or a medical social worker usually acts as the salesperson. This person is fully aware of the home health agencies and the services they provide. When arranging to discharge a patient, then, the hospital coordinator determines if the patient will need aftercare at home and appropriately refers the patient to the agency. The hospital coordinator seeks out the consumer/patient who needs services. Thus, health services are promoted by the utilization of personal selling.[14]

The marketing plan must devise a way for the agency to deliver its services. Home health care agencies generally have a staff that provides health services to the consumer. For example, home care agencies have a service team that furnishes direct care to patients through physicians, nurses, medical social workers, therapists, nutritionists, housekeepers, etc. The agencies are the producer-providers that distribute services through the service team and on to the consumer (the patient).[15]

This marketing plan is used to address the segment of the population in immediate need of services. Most of these consumers were previously institutionalized and aware of their other alternative—to receive care at home. But what about the segment of the market for whom no immediate need exists? In marketing the concept of home health care it is important that all segments of the market be reached, for home care is a service that one may not be in need of now but may want to utilize in the future. In other words, the market plan should be directed to the entire population because everyone may potentially need home care. Because the marketing plan has been directed mainly at the market in need of the services, some agencies have been underutilized and underdeveloped. As a result, in order to serve long-run needs, the market must be changed so that potential users are knowledgeable of the services available to them.[16] Accordingly, the market plan must be reorganized to encompass the group between twenty-five and fifty-five years old as well. The best approach to extend services to those with no immediate need is through education. A strong educational campaign will reduce the underuse of services due to lack of awareness and will encourage the use of this valuable health care delivery mode. To attract the attention of this age group, an education program should attempt to make them aware of the agency's services. One way to do this is to promote the capabilities of the agency as a provider. An introductory letter explaining the agency's services is one method of educating the market about available options to institutional care.[17]

Another method is through a slide program or film. Home health care dealers seldom use audiovisual presentations to advertise themselves to potential customers and referral sources. But films have a great impact on potential home care customers. They are usually targeted to health professionals: physicians, nurses, therapists, hospital administrators, etc. Part of the film will depict the hospital setting, demonstrating how the physicians, therapists, and discharge planners coordinate a plan for removing patients from the hospital and into a home environment. The second part of the film will show the patients' life at home, including the materials they use and the support personnel who regularly assist them. Films are also a good marketing tool for reinforcing the necessity of advanced planning in sending a patient home. After seeing the film, hospital personnel and physicians should be more inclined to send referrals and business to the agency, because the film shows that home care providers know what they are doing and that they care about the patient and do the best for everyone. These promotional channels educate the market, and as a result can lead to an effort to expand services into a community not formerly serviced — the group between twenty-five and fifty-five years old.[18]

Once the market has been educated about home care, what is available and what it has to offer them, other tools of marketing in the area of public relations can be used to sell the concept of home care. A speakers' bureau will continue to provide information about the services available and increase the agency's credibility. Brochures are another marketing tool designed to meet the competitive market. They contain information that supports home care as opposed to institutional care. Another technique is to capitalize on events that "gain the maximum media coverage." For example, a health fair sponsored by the agency may receive radio time and space for newspaper advertisements. Positive interaction within the community and building strong public relations will increase the acceptance of the agency. Above all, high visibility of the agency is the key to successfully marketing a service.[19]

## The Purpose of Marketing Incentives

Why should the producer care to sell the services? Obviously, there is an urgent need to find alternatives to hospital health care, but why home health care? Home care is very desirable and viewed as a marketable product worth selling due to the incentive it offers. Home health care offers many benefits over institutional care.

### Sociological Benefits
Until recently, community services were fragmented and health and social services were widely dispersed. Most of the people in need of these home health care services were unable to find these services, and since they were so dispersed, it was difficult to arrange for the appropriate combination of services. After seeking and compiling these

services, they had to find various payment sources to finance them. This fragmentation reduces the efficiency and effectiveness of services and forces people to depend on institutions for comprehensive services. The system is changing, however, and society is moving back toward a coordinated home health care delivery system. Instead of patients seeking their own services, the delivery of home health care involves many people, including service providers and third-party payers who work together to provide home care — hospitals, skilled nursing facilities, and physicians combine their services and make them accessible to the individual.[20]

### Psychological Benefits

Patients who are cared for in hospitals or nursing homes are cut off from normal home life and the closeness of family and friends. Home care enhances patients' lives by allowing them to stay in a familiar environment surrounded by loving family members who want to help care for them. When patients are at home with those who love and care for one another, they have a greater chance of recovering emotionally. In addition, family support enables the patient to "mobilize all of the physical and psychological resources to cope with stress and to cooperate in rehabilitation." The family is also a useful element in therapy. The family members know and understand the patient's needs and interests and can usually arrange activities that are fulfilling and gratifying, especially when other members participate. At home patients' needs are respected. They are free to do things as they please. This range of choices makes recovery at home easier. Also, patients are able to gain a sense of selfhood at home because they are able to make choices that reflect their self-image, e.g., choosing what clothes to wear. Every opportunity for change and choice allows patients to feel as though they are acting for themselves and have control over their lives. Psychologically, this helps patients gain confidence in themselves and cope with their illness.[21]

### Economic Benefits

Hospital costs are rising rapidly and as a result health care consumers are looking for less expensive alternatives to institutional care. Illness and treatment can be a severe financial burden, which is likely to deplete a large portion of the family's income. Since institutional care involves sociological and psychological costs as well as high economic costs, consumers are turning to home care, which is less expensive and offers psychological and social benefits. In today's society, cost saving — without a loss of quality of care — is an important asset.

Even though the social utility of expanded home health care is highly desirable, there is a potentially negative aspect: "social utility must be balanced with cost considerations." The methods used to finance home care today include: direct payments, voluntary prepayment mechanisms, compulsory prepayment mechanisms, tax funds, and private philanthropy. Before home care can be considered for reimbursement, the cost of organized home care must be determined and standardized. The financial situation of many states will make them very cautious about the ultimate cost of expanded home health care and whether they can afford to reimburse for home care services. The main focus, then, will be on quality assurance and control of utilization. Once the form of reimbursement has been changed, home care will be an extremely marketable concept.

*Medicare*

The reimbursement system for comprehensive home health services greatly influences the development of the present health care system — institutional care. Third-party payers and other forms of reimbursement — Medicare and Medicaid — need to be changed to promote home care and meet the demands of the consumer. At this time, although home care is less expensive, forms of reimbursement favor institutional care, and until this is changed, people will continue to use services that are reimbursable.[23]

Payment for aftercare services has not kept up with the need, and as a result, patients remain in the hospital for longer periods of time than they need to. Less than half of the people under sixty-five are covered by health insurance for home care mainly because insurance benefits do not include home care. Under Medicare, the elderly may receive up to one hundred visits at home by a nurse or other skilled health professional if they satisfy the necessary conditions. These restrictions make very few people eligible for home health benefits and encourage the use of hospitals. For example, one condition states they may receive benefits if "they have been in the hospital three days excluding the day of discharge." Eliminating this requirement alone would presumably discourage beneficiaries, who only need home care, to seek costly hospitalization. Changing Medicare benefits would increase the marketability of the concept of home care. By eliminating restrictive barriers, the provider would encourage the use of home health care. Similarly, changing the "skilled" requirement would facilitate the provision of home health care, since many people do not require skilled care. Many patients require services, but no skilled care, to minimize deterioration in functioning. These services could delay or prevent the need for more costly services later on if this condition were changed. Therefore, it would be more cost-effective if services were matched with need. The guidelines of Medicare benefit only those in institutions, but could have a widespread effect on the entire health care delivery system if the conditions were not as restrictive. It would also enable people with minor needs to acquire services before it is too late and they are institutionalized. Changes in Medicare would make home care a very marketable alternative.[24]

## Medicaid

The same is true of Medicaid as for Medicare. Medicaid gives little encouragement to the development of home care. It is a state system that reimburses those who cannot pay their medical bills. There are conditions one must meet to become a candidate for reimbursement. Medicaid pays the medical bills for those people whose income is below levels established by law. This is a very restrictive requirement especially for those patients who have a healthy spouse and family; to be eligible, most of the financial resources have to be used up, which would leave the family impoverished.[25] As a result, unless the requirements for receiving Medicaid change, home care will be a service many potential consumers cannot afford.

## Problems in Marketing

When marketing a product or service, it is essential that providers know the problems they will encounter ahead of time so they will be easier to face. The financial problems involved in reimbursement have already been examined, but there are many more. For example, a major problem in gaining support for home care is the lack of uniform standards and ways to regulate quality of care given at home.[26] Consumers like to have knowledge of what it is they are purchasing, so unless the provider demonstrates the effectiveness of home care it will be a difficult concept to sell. Most of the problems can be attributed to lack of knowledge of home health care. The true role of home health care has not been well understood or sold to the population. The solution is to *educate the consumer*. Many hospital days could be saved by more prompt utilization of home health care.

Another major problem is changing the present health care delivery system. Medicare and Medicaid have created multibillion-dollar sources of federal dollars that support institutional care. Hospitals and physicians have a powerful incentive to keep things as they are. Why send patients home, if the hospital can make a profit by keeping them longer? A hospital that is not full is reluctant to discharge a low-cost-for-care patient. It is also in the physician's best interest to keep the hospital full. The medical community does not support home care because it is viewed as competition. Home health agencies offer the same services a hospital provides, but at a lower price. Although it will be difficult to change physicians' attitudes, agencies should meet with physicians in a cooperative effort to indicate how home health care can serve as "an extension of his concern for the patient." Once physicians are informed, one hopes they will advertise or promote home care and refer patients to agencies to receive care.[27]

In the long run, home health care will actually save money by keeping people out of hospitals and nursing homes, which are the most expensive forms of care. Politicians, who make policy decisions concerning financing of home care, are concerned with accountability and the short term — the time between now and the next election. Quality of care in homes appears to be good, although standards and levels of performance vary widely. Politicians, if they support home care, are accountable to consumers, health providers, and the community. They are accountable to the consumer to ensure that the services are available and utilized. There is also a concern with home health providers delivering the services they advertise.

When a major issue such as quality is involved, and there is a lack of knowledge in this area, it is difficult to make changes in how home health care services are delivered. All people involved in policy decisions concerning health care delivery should be educated. Major changes are not necessary now, but even small policy shifts will be enough to display the marketability of home care.

The final problem in marketing home care is selling it to the caretaker. Not only does a disease drain the patient's physical and emotional resources, but also the family's resources. In many cases the illness changes the pattern of the family's life. Patient care involves both mental and physical preparation for meeting immediate and chronic care needs. Mental preparation includes considering the patient and understanding how a doctor thinks about a patient and how the doctor orders care. Physical preparation involves collecting necessary equipment and organizing it in the best way possible. This means that the caretaker may be totally tied down. In this case, it may be difficult to convince the caretaker that home care is the best method of health care delivery. The provider must, then, especially sell the benefits of home care to the caretaker.[28]

## Conclusion

Hospitals are cold and impersonal and have long been thought of as places where people go to die. The home, on the other hand, is a warm and secure place where a person lives. When given a choice, it is the consumer who must decide what mode of health care delivery to use. Providers marketing home care must convince the consumer that care in a general hospital is not only expensive but unsuited to the medical, emotional, and social needs of many patients.[29] In other words, providers must promote the advantages of home care over institutional care. Providers stress the reasons for purchasing home care. One reason for home care is the spiraling cost of hospitalization; home care is much less expensive. Also, patients are often happier and respond more readily to treatment in a familiar environment. If there is a shortage of hospital beds or if hospitals and doctors are widely scattered and not readily available, home care may be necessary. Home care offers many benefits that make it a desirable service for the consumer to purchase.

There are several factors that influence an individual's choice of home care. Home care does not mean that medical help is rejected; in fact, medical services are a major provider of home care.[30] Ultimately, the doctor decides if a patient needs home care; but others are involved as well. Home health care requires great cooperation from the patient and even greater demands on the family. As a result, there are two important factors in deciding on home care: what the patient wants, because recovery and quality of life during illness depend on mental attitude; and what the family wants and can realistically provide. The family must evaluate strengths and weaknesses in time available for care, financial assets and health care benefits, and the emotional attitude about the illness. To provide home care the family priorities have to be evaluated. Once this has been done and the options have been evaluated, a decision can be made. Successful marketing of the concept of home health care will show that home health care is an appealing service.

# 17

## CONCLUDING
## THOUGHTS

A t some point in their lives, most human beings ponder the question "How long and how well will I live?" Although the answer to this question is unknown to most of us, our ideas on how we should live and die are strongly influenced by prevailing social attitudes and practices.

Our constant, though often involuntary, interaction with the bureaucracies of our society has rendered us vulnerable to institutional domination and control of our lives.[1]

Needless to say, this encourages the submissiveness that immobilizes people and limits their self-reliance and independence. Service sectors, in particular, often pursue internal objectives that are not in the public interest.[2] Because most institutions are unlikely to advertise alternatives to their services, the consumer is usually left uninformed and incapable of making rational choices.

Thus, consumers are forced into situations over which they have no control, having relinquished it to the "authorities" upon entering the system. This is the first step in the gradual process of degrading an individual's integrity and self-determination. People are not expected to reject or question services provided by the institution, even if it becomes apparent that those services are inadequate and/or inappropriate.

One of the most illustrative examples of this phenomenon is the inability of modern medical institutions to provide adequate care for the terminally ill.[3] In this chapter, I will address the qualitative aspect of institutional care for the dying and expose the effects of its inadequacies on dying patients and their families. I will then focus on the potential of home care for reforming these inadequacies and providing a feasible and desirable alternative to the hospital experience. The benefits of this type of care to patients and their families will be discussed, in addition to a few of the limitations. In most instances, home care has the potential to address issues long neglected by the hospital, issues that undermine the quality of care available to patients and their families. A brief discussion of traditional methods of caring is now in order.

Despite advances in medical and technical competence, the medical institution has yet to find a cure for diseases diagnosed as "chronic."[4] Yet patients found to have these diseases are still placed under the auspices of care-oriented, technology-based systems, where they are treated with modern drugs and equipment that increase the quantity of their lives while decreasing the quality.

Because terminal diseases such as cancer are not "treatable" in the usual sense, the hospital staff eventually loses interest in the dying patient. Low value is placed on providing quality care for terminal patients; cancer units are often found in the oldest and least accessible part of a hospital. Decisions concerning the extent and type of care usually reflect the physician's economic interests rather than attempts to cater to the patient's needs. Thus, the quality of care comes to be determined independently of its outcomes and becomes a factor of the amount of expensive equipment and techniques used in treatment. The fact is that most hospitals are money-making institutions and cannot realistically be expected to provide the type of care a dying patient needs. The hospital is a completely inappropriate place for the dying, and this is easily deduced from its therapeutic orientation; hospital staffs are trained to cure the living, not care for the dying.[5]

The hospital is not only uninterested in the needs of dying patients, it does not have the resources to treat them. Institutions, for purposes of "efficiency," demand that individuals succumb to their authority even if this discourages attention directed at the nonmedical needs of the patient. For all practical purposes, patients are expected to adopt a completely submissive and accepting attitude toward the range of hospital procedures that have been designated as appropriate for the particular "condition." All aspects of treatment are beyond the patient's control, and this is perceived as one of the most unbearable aspects of hospitalization. Dealing with a terminal illness requires much readjustment on the part of patients in an institution that undermines their autonomy so that it can produce its commodities "efficiently."[6]

The patient pays a high price for this efficient care, such as having to endure pain until caregivers decide medication is needed. Experts in palliative care maintain that "PRN" or "as needed" administration of pain medication is inappropriate in the treatment of chronic pain. The patient should not be subjected to caregivers' interpretation of the "right" time to relieve pain. This practice, quite common in hospitals, is depersonalizing and inhumane.[7]

Another negative aspect of hospitalization is the physical setup of the rooms, which discourages visitors by limiting space and sitting room. Patients are separated from those around them by high-rise bed apparatus and hospital equipment, in addition to being allowed only limited time for interaction with loved ones. Needless to say, these factors tend to increase patient anxiety, and consequently patients tend to report more pain in hospitals than they do at home. Although hospitals can and do treat pain, their neglect of its contributing factors and of the emotional needs of their patients decreases the overall quality of their care. In fact, most of the real needs of a dying person are not "treatable" in a hospital. Although people have individual needs, a few concerns are shared by most dying people:

- a sense of urgency to complete one's life goals due to temporal restrictions
- loss of control and forced dependency
- sense of isolation
- need to "come to terms" with life[8]

Although these concerns do not stem from being institutionalized, they are compounded by interaction with a philosophy that is antithetical to their needs.

The patient is not the only victim of institutional inadequacy; in fact it is often more difficult for the family members to deal with the limitations of hospital-based care. This is primarily due to their total lack of control over the patient's treatment and activities. In addition, hospitals cannot and do not promote complete resolution of the grief process. Ultimately, it means the deterioration of the physical and mental health of patients and their families.

This is supported by Dr. Robert Mendelsohn, author of *Confessions of a Medical Heretic,* who states in his book that "for a doctor to succeed, he must impose his ethics and beliefs in place of the family's. Not only don't doctors share feelings, cultures, and traditions, they also don't care what happens. If a patient dies, it's not a tragedy because he/she is a patient."

Hospitals tend to disrupt family roles and structures by severely undermining their autonomy. Family members are often unaware of their right to intervene or protest and must therefore submit to hospital measures for lack of alternatives. When dying people are put into institutions, there is often little consideration given to the coping needs of their families. A social support network has usually not been established, nor is it likely one will develop within the hospital. In spite of this, family members are virtually ignored in most hospital situations. Their intervention is usually considered unimportant and they are seen as an appendage of the patient that must be tolerated and controlled. Time is not allotted for family care, so the final days in a person's life are spent under hospital jurisdiction, with inadequate attention to the family unit. It is not difficult to understand the growing dissatisfaction with the hospital as a place for dying. The idea that it is more humane to let the dying succumb to their illness, without heroic, life-prolonging intervention, has become more accepted and even welcomed. An alternative that has reemerged is the home care program, which transfers the locus of care from the hospital to the home. There are certain prerequisites to the home care alternative:

• "Care-oriented" treatment has been discounted, with an emphasis on care
  • patient expresses desire to be at home
  • family expresses desire to bring patient home
  • family recognizes their ability to care for patient
  • a nurse willing to be on call twenty-four hours a day
  • a physician needed as a consultant[9]

The philosophy of this care revolves around the desire to maintain individual and family integrity and self-determination. This is hardly possible when both are undermined by the imposition of hospital procedures.

If the claim were verified that an individual has the right to self-determination in matters of life and death and he or she chose to live, we would expect others to respect this choice and, if possible, help to protect this person's life. Similarly, if an individual chose to die, we should consider it a duty to assist that person's dying.[10]

This does not only involve controlling the physical symptoms of dying, but also attending to the emotional and spiritual needs of the dying, which are just as, if not more, important. It is important to remember the difference between physical and psychological dependence. Patients can be totally dependent on others for physical care and yet maintain their autonomy.[11] This means the patient must have a voice in decisions and an ability to influence the timing and type of activities, what communication occurs, and the setup of the immediate environment. This means that a nurse cannot walk into a patient's room at any hour to administer medication or perform a treatment without the patient's consent.

There are a variety of advantages that home care can offer to the individual patient. Once basic fears of isolation and dependence are alleviated, it becomes easier for the patient to confront and deal with the "other" issues of dying; any degree of control, security, and comfort will decrease patient anxiety.

Home care permits many opportunities for providing an individualized approach to the provision of care. One such example is the preparation of food. Although this might not seem to be an issue, it is actually a necessity in terms of ensuring optimal nutritional intake. Contrast this to the hospital, where, in the words of Norman Cousins, author of *Anatomy of an Illness*, "Perhaps the most serious failure was in the area of nutrition. It was not just that the meals were poorly balanced, what was inexcusable to me was the profusion of processed foods, some of which contained preservatives or harmful dyes. White bread was offered with every meal. Vegetables were often over-cooked and thus deprived of much of their nutritional value."[12] Today, there is little dispute over the fact that diet is crucial to health and well-being; this should not be neglected in the care of dying people.

Another advantage of home care is that it allows individuals to maintain a "place" in their family structure. They are surrounded by their loved ones in a setting that is familiar and safe to them. This enables them to look around and see what their existence has meant, to observe their lives in context. Peace of mind is possible only if the patient is relaxed and able to confront the difficult issues of dying. Dying patients experience an awareness of their finitude, and this precipitates a "life review" of previous experiences in an attempt to maintain a sense of continuity over time. Patients, upon experiencing this life review, attempt to make sense of their stories so that their lives retain meaning.[13]

Other problems that need attention are the resolution and relationships of unmet goals. The individual living within an institution has little opportunity to resolve family conflicts because family members are discouraged from spending time at the hospital. Caring for the patient at home makes the resolution of such relationship problems more likely.

A final problem involves the resolution of unmet goals. This can be a source of frustration and anxiety. Hospital personnel obviously have no time to help patients examine alternative approaches to pursue their goals. Once again, the family members in a home care situation can address this issue by facilitating identification of these goals and helping the patient either achieve his or her goals or develop more pressing ones.[14]

If persons caring for a dying individual exhibit a desire to provide the type of attentive care he or she needs, a great contribution would have been made toward increasing the quality of their limited time. One aspect of this attentive care is ensuring patient awareness of the environment; knowing what to expect provides predictability, which is therapeutic to the disrupted and unpredictable lifestyle the patient and family have had to endure prior to the onset of home care. A daily schedule of activities also reduces patient dependence because he or she will not make demands if it is known when demands will be attended to. A system of scheduling such things as baths, medication, and meals will provide family members with a cooperative system that is predictable to the patient and serves to distribute responsibility of care among them.[15]

A dying person must be allowed to maintain his or her self-care activities until physically unable to do so. A typical day might begin with a family member bringing the patient the necessary equipment to wash and freshen up. Conditions permitting, a change of environment is recommended during the day time when energy is high and pain lowest.[16] A ride in a wheelchair or nap in the garden has unique psychological benefits.

Boredom also becomes a problem at the hospital since it is not equipped for long-term stays. Patients often lie in bed all day with few entertainment possibilities. At home, the potential for alleviating this problem is greatly increased. The day can be broken up into small activities, such as breakfast, washing up, a wheelchair ride, a meditation session, a massage, card playing, an afternoon discussion — all of which give the patient something to look forward to.[17] Many patients express the desire to be outdoors as much as possible. As long as wheelchair rides or walks are physically possible, they can and should be included in a home care program.

At some point, dying undermines an individual's ability to make decisions for him or herself. As adults, we need to make independent choices, and caretakers must therefore make an effort to provide the most opportunity for patients to feel that their input counts. Home care also provides the potential for complete control of pain medication. While hospitalized, patients are structured by the hospital's timetable for administration of pain medication. Often patients needlessly suffer in hospitals while waiting for relief. The secret of pain control is to administer medication at definite intervals, "to prevent pain from occurring rather than controlling it once it is present."[18] This is only possible at home because hospitals continue to operate under "PRN," "as needed," guidelines. Of course, it is necessary for the family and nurse-aide to be given complete flexibility in pain management by the physician.

A discussion of the advantages of home care for individuals cannot be complete without consideration of the advantages extended to their families. The family and patient who choose to go through the dying experience together and at home tend to be more well adjusted to their fate than their hospitalized counterparts.[19] The experience tends to bond families under circumstances that are usually divisive. This has many positive implications for the family, including the possibility of alleviating guilt often experienced in such situations. The family is given the opportunity to do everything "humanly possible" to care for their loved one, making his or her dying a family experience.

The family is not separated and its structure is maintained within a familiar environment. Different members of the family are given specific responsibilities in the "caregiving," and this creates a feeling of closeness and solidarity among them. The dramatic change in their lives is made easier when shared.

According to Stephen and Andrea Levine, codirectors at the Dying Project in New Mexico, there are a few things that will help make the experience easier for patients and their families. Some of these include:

- a cassette recorder for music and meditation
- a bedside bell
- plastic bedpan
- daily baths
- massage
- blender for liquid meals
- hot plate
- side rails on bed
- available pain medication
- bed in living room
- strong supportive measures[20]

Although the parents are the primary caregivers in a home care situation, a nurse or "home aide" is helpful in most circumstances to provide assistance, support, and the type of professional expertise that facilitates communication in difficult situations. During the dying process, patients need to have at least one person with whom continuous, meaningful communication is possible. Although communication of this type does occur between the patient and family, it might not provide the patient with the same benefits that an objective, experienced listener offers.[21]

A nurse can sometimes help a patient adopt more effective coping strategies by demonstrating acceptance, setting reasonable limits, and establishing trust by being reliable about providing care and making it easier for the family to work within their limited framework.[22]

Patients can express the total range of their feelings to the nurse without fear of causing the emotional impact a family member might experience. This is important because otherwise feelings would be directed inward or expressed through behavior patterns. If necessary, a nurse can guide patients and their families in times of crisis by maintaining open channels of communication.

Home care encourages the family to learn from and change with their experience by giving them the responsibility of providing care.

Family members are taught necessary medical techniques and are exposed to new ideas and philosophies of life. The last stages of life should not be seen as a defeat but rather as a time for life's fulfillment, not a time of negation but one with potential for positive achievement.[23] Care of the dying demands that everything be done to enable patients to live fully until they die. The time at home can be a very powerful bonding experience. It is often a time of resolving family differences and reaffirming their love for each other. By confronting their lives without their loved one and making appropriate plans for the future, they maintain the continuity of life.

As with any type of care, there exist a few limitations and drawbacks to caring for a dying person at home. The most significant are the emotional and physical strain placed on the family. Their needs are often abandoned in favor of providing comfort for the dying patient. Family goals and future plans are also abandoned and activities revolve around the patient. This can be unhealthy in both the short- and long-term perspective. Resentment toward the patient for forcing the family to disrupt their old lifestyle and adjust to their new one is increased when the patient has many siblings. This resentment can be expressed in destructive ways and will not promote grief resolution. In the long run, when family goals are abandoned it leaves the family with no sense of closure or continuity.

Caring for a patient twenty-four hours a day often results in physical exhaustion. Sleep can become a luxury, and meeting personal needs takes on secondary importance. A type of pain is experienced if tension is allowed to mount and there is no outlet for family mem-bers.[24] Outside contact is essential, but what often happens in home-care situations (especially advanced ones) is the gradual "closing in" of the home to outsiders. This is potentially harmful to the patient because he or she will be likely to perceive his or her illness as causing the disruption and trouble the family is experiencing.

It is clear that terminal illness within a family usually brings about experiences that are allowed to be psychologically and socially destructive to patients and their families. These same experiences, however, can be viewed in a positive way by both.

During the dying process, many patients begin to consider the meaning of their lives in terms of a greater whole. It seems to be a time when many dying people feel as though they truly appreciate and understand life for the first time. People begin to look into their own hearts and the eyes of their loved ones and often find, as most of us would, that these aren't places we've looked deeply enough in the past. This is why dying people seem to extract from life all it has to offer. In the words of one dying man, "We're such fools, aren't we? We spend so much time polishing our personalities, strengthening our bodies, keeping our social positions, trying to achieve this and that. We make such a serious business of it all. But now that I can no longer do the things I thought were so important, I have so much love for so many things. I'm discovering a place inside myself I'd never looked at, never knew. None of the praise I received in the past brought me half the satisfaction I experience right now from just being."[25]

From this, we can see the dying can experience growth from what they face. It is we, the living, who can learn from them. The dying teach us that the real tragedy of life is not dying, or death, but rather the waste of life on superficial relationships and meaningless pursuits.

We have learned to equate living well with material acquisition and never pause to ponder the meaning of our life. We have also learned to deny death and are therefore unprepared for it. The dying teach us that it is all right to die, that it is an unavoidable and natural part of life. They teach us that it is often the living who close themelves off to life, not the dying. It is these people who never develop an acceptance and awareness of life who will experience death with great struggle and horror.[26]

This need not be the case. Unfortunately, our society has consistently denied death, and for this reason medical institutions have become the "acceptable" place to die. This trend has proven detrimental to patients, argues Ivan Illich, author of *Medical Nemesis*. He writes, "Medicine unquestionably injures more than it cures — not just through crude technology but essentially because it has stripped patients of the tools to take care of themselves." Illich refers to this as "social introgenesis." The medical institutions' monopoly over health as a good is matched by its "control" over death. A paradox emerges: medicine deals in disease by selling units of health and deals with death by selling units of life. In neither case is the patient given responsibility for the results. The hospital experience, therefore, is anything but conducive to meeting the real needs of dying patients and their families. The opportunity for growth and positive experience is greatly decreased.[27]

This is the area most dramatically affected by a home care program. The commitment to go through the experience as a family unit, within a home, although not without its hardships, has the potential of fulfillment that no institution could provide. It is a reaffirmation of the continuity of life and provides a wholistic view of an otherwise fragmented social reality. The highly personalized aspect of home care will increase the likelihood that people will die in a manner congruent with their previous lifestyle. It means dying patients will get the respect they deserve and the unique care they require. In addition, home care makes it possible for family members to experience growth and insight from what they have shared. Perhaps the greatest gift the dying have to offer us is the realization that we do not have to wait until we have a terminal illness to look at our lives and decide if we are realizing the potential of our humanity.

# NOTES

## Chapter 1 / Introduction to Home Health Care

1. Edith Wensley, *Nursing Service Without Walls: A Call to Action to All Communities Coast to Coast* (New York: National League for Nursing, 1963), pp. 15–16.

2. Helen M. F. Bartholomew, "Home Care Nursing: The Consumer's Perception" (M.A. diss., University of Arizona, 1976), p. 37.

3. Valerie LaPorte and Jeffrey Rubin, eds., *Reform and Regulation in Long Term Care* (New York: Praeger Publishers, 1979), pp. 36–37.

4. Joseph A. Papsidero, Sidney Katz, Sr., Mary Honora Kroger, and C. Amechi Abpom, eds., *Chance for Change: Implications of a Chronic Disease Module Study* (Lansing: Michigan State University Press, 1979), p. 103.

5. Elizabeth R. Prichard, Jean Collard, Janet Starr, Josephine A. Lockwood, Austin H. Kutscher, and Irene B. Seeland, eds., *Home Care: Living with Dying* (New York: Columbia University Press, 1979), p. 137.

6. Prichard, p. 138.

7. C. Carl Pegels, "Institutional v. Noninstitutional Care for the Elderly," *Journal of Health Politics, Policy and Law* 5, no. 2 (1980):209.

8. Prichard, p. 17.

9. Pegels, p. 206.

10. Papsidero, p. 11.

11. James J. Callahan, Jr., and Stanley S. Wallack, eds., *Reforming the Long Term Care System* (Lexington, Mass.: D.C. Heath and Co., 1981), pp. 14 and 17.

12. Ibid., p. 14.

13. LaPorte, pp. 36–37.

14. Callahan, pp. 38–39.

15. Papsidero, p. 12.

16. Ibid., p. 17.

17. Pegels, p. 210.

18. Ibid.

19. Cynthia Anderson, "Home or Nursing Home? Let the Elderly Patient Decide," *American Journal of Nursing* 79, no. 8 (1979):1148.

20. Mary E. Laver and Bruce M. Camitta, "Home Care for Dying Children: A Nursing Model," *The Journal of Pediatrics* 97, no. 6 (1980):1034.

21. Maureen O'Brien Flaherty, *The Care of the Elderly Person: A Guide for the Licensed Practical Nurse* (St. Louis: C.V. Mosby Co., 1980), pp. 150–51.

22. James A. Koncel, "Home Health Care Can Be Reimbursed," *Hospitals* 53, no. 20 (1979):44–45.

23. National League for Nursing, *Accreditation of Home Health Agencies and Community Nursing Services* (National League for Nursing, publication no. 21-1612, 1976).

24. Judith Meltzer, Frank Farrow, and Harold Richman, eds., *Policy Options in Long Term Care* (Chicago: University of Chicago Press, 1981), pp. 14–17.

## Chapter 2 / The History of Home Health Care

1. Earland Cyrus, "A Historical Perspective on Home Health Care," in *Home Care: Living with Dying,* ed. Elizabeth R. Prichard et al. (New York: Columbia University Press, 1979), p. 12.

2. Jane Emmert Stewart, *Home Health Care* (St. Louis: C.V. Mosby Co., 1978), p. 50.

3. Ibid., p. 65.

4. Nancy Robinson, *"The Homemaker–Home Health Aide," The Issue Is Leadership* (New York: National League for Nursing, 1975), p. 85; Stewart, pp. 90–91.

5. Stewart, p. 92.

6. Ibid., p. 94.

7. Celia Moss Hailperin, "Twenty-Five Years of Home Care Services," *Home Care: Living with Dying,* p. 137.

8. C. R. Ryder, *Changing Patterns in Home Care* (Arlington, Va.: Department of Health, Education, and Welfare, 1967).

9. Hailperin, p. 137.

10. Cyrus, p. 13.

11. Ibid.

12. Hailperin, p. 138.

13. Stewart, p. 20.

14. J. J. Hanlon and George E. Pickett, *Public Health Administration*

*and Practice* (St. Louis: C.V. Mosby Co., 1974), p. 645; Catherine Tinkham and Eleanor F. Voorhies, *Community Health Nursing: Evolution and Process* (New York: Appleton-Century-Crofts, 1977), pp. 18–20.

15. Tinkham and Voorhies, pp. 18–20; Hanlon and Pickett, p. 645.

16. Stewart, p. 20.

17. Cyrus, pp. 13–14.

18. Ibid., p. 14.

19. Gertrude Sturges, "Organized Medical Care of the Sick in Their Homes," *The Hospital Survey for New York* (New York: United Hospital Fund, 1937), p. 820; New York City Charter (New York: City Record Office, 1951).

20. F. Jenson, J. G. Weisbotten, and M. A. Thomas, *Medical Care of the Discharged Hospital Patient* (New York: Commonwealth Fund, 1944; republished by Harvard University Press, Cambridge, Mass.).

21. Hospital Council of Greater New York, *Organized Home Medical Care in New York City* (New York: Harvard University Press, 1956), p. 346, Appendix A.

22. Hailperin, p. 140.

23. Ibid.

24. Robert J. Myers, *Medicare* (Illinois: McCahan Foundation, 1970), pp. 62–63; Stewart, pp. 97–99.

25. Stewart, p. 97.

26. Ibid.

27. Ibid.

28. Ibid., pp. 111–12.

29. Ibid., p. 20.

30. Ibid., pp. 149–51.

31. Ibid., pp. 12–13.

32. Ibid., p. 13.

**Chapter 3 / Legislation and Home Care Services, 1935–1982**

1. Florence A. Wilson and Duncan Newhauser, *Health Services in the United States* (Cambridge, Mass.: Ballinger Publishing Co., 1982), p. 168.

2. Ibid., p. 170.

3. Ibid., p. 172; Margaret Greenfield, *Medicare and Medicaid: The 1965 and 1967 Social Security Amendments* (California: Institute of Governmental Studies, 1968), p. 71.

4. Ibid., p. 47.

5. Wilson, p. 307; Greenfield, p. 7.

6. Wilson, p. 313.

7. Ibid.

8. Ibid., p. 314.

9. Greenfield, p. 7.

10. *Trends Affecting the U. S. Health Care System* (Massachusetts: Cambridge Research Institute, 1976), p. 121.

11. Greenfield, p. 12; Robert J. Meyers, *Medicare* (Pennsylvania: McCahan Foundation, 1970), p. 114.

12. Carol J. Lundberg, "Home Care Legislation: New Tax Bill Mandates Changes for H.H.A.'s," *Hospitals* 56, no. 21 (1982):81.

13. Ibid., p. 81.

14. Meyers, p. 223.

15. Wilson, p. 180.

16. Douglas R. Mackintosh, *Systems of Health Care* (Boulder: Westview Press, 1978), p. 104.

17. Philip H. Abelson, ed., *Health Care Regulations: Economics, Ethics, Practices* (Washington, D.C.: American Association for the Advancement of Science, 1978), p.106.

18. Mackintosh, p. 101.

19. Ibid., pp. 102–3.

20. Wilson, p. 183.

21. Ibid., p. 193.

22. Janice M. Caldwell, "Home Care: Utilizing Resources to Develop Home Care," *Hospitals* 56, no. 21 (1982):68.

23. Ibid.

24. Judith A. Collins, "Medicare and Medicaid: Cuts and Concerns," *Geriatrics* 37, no. 1 (1982):24 and 34.

25. Ibid., p.38.

26. "Respite Care Meets a Desperate Need for Many Families," *Aging* 337 (1983):31.

27. Caterine Frasca, "Home Health Care Program Offers Comprehensive Services," *Hospitals* 55, no.6 (1981):39–42.

## Chapter 4 / The Psychological Effects of Home Care

1. L. B. Murphy, *The Home Hospital: How a Family Can Cope with Catastrophic Illness* (New York: Basic Books, 1982), p. 5.

2. Ibid., pp. 9, 12, and 14.

3. Patricia A. Kennedy, *Dying at Home with Cancer* (Springfield, Ill.: Charles C. Thomas, 1982), p. 7; Murphy, pp. 13–14.

4. Murphy, p. 155.

5. Ibid., pp. 15–17 and 149–50.

6. David Agle, "Home Care—Psychological Benefits and Hazards," *Scandinavian Journal of Hematology* 30 (1977):66–69.

7. Judy Henri, "An Alternative to Institutionalization," *The Gerontologist* 20, no. 4 (1980): 418-20.

8. Genrose J. Alfano, "There Are No Routine Patients." *American Journal of Nursing* 75, no. 10 (1975:1805; Mildred Horn, "Hospital-Based Home Care," *American Journal of Nursing* 75, no. 10 (1975):1811.

9. S. Wolk, and S. Telleen, "Psychological and Social Correlates of Life Satisfaction as a Function of Residential Constraint," *Journal of Gerontology* 31, no. 1 (1976):89.

10. Michael Jospe et al., eds., *Psycholical Factors in Health Care: A Practitioner's Manual* (Lexington, Mass.: D. C. Heath and Co., 1980), p. 218.

11. Alfano, p. 1806; Susan L. Huges, "Home Health Monitoring," *Hospitals* 56, no. 1 (1982):77.

12. I. M. Burnside, "Health Care of the Confused Elderly at Home," *Nursing Clinics of North America* 15, no. 2 (1980):398.

13. Henri, pp. 418-20.

14. M. J. Hennessey and B. Gorenberg, "The Significance and Impact of the Home Care of an Older Adult," *Nursing Clinics of North America* 15, no. 2 (1980):359.

15. Robert Buckingham, "Public Health Policy and Terminal Care," *The Arizona Review* 29, no. 2 (1980), pp. 18-19; Kennedy, p. 7-10; Robert Buckingham, "Hospice Care in the United States—The Process Begins," *OMEGA* 13, no. 2 (1982-83):161.

16. Ida M. Martinson et al., "Home Care for Children Dying of Cancer," *Pediatrics* 62, no. 1 (1978):106; Robert Buckingham, *A Special Kind of Love: Care of the Dying Child* (New York: Continuum, 1983), p. 66.

17. Ida Martinson et al., "When the Patient Is Dying: Home Care for the Child," *American Journal of Nursing* 77, no. 11 (1977):1817; Buckingham, *A Special Kind of Love*, p. 69.

18. Martinson, "When the Patient," p. 1817.

19. Buckingham, *A Special Kind of Love*, pp. 69-70.

20. Anne J. Davis, "Disability, Home Care and the Care-Taking Role in the Family Life," *Journal of Advanced Nursing* 5 (1980):479 and 481.

21. M. R. Lipp, *Respectful Treatment: The Human Side of Medical Care* (New York: Harper and Row, 1977), p. 174; Burnside, p. 392.

22. Murphy, pp. 17 and 272; Vida Goldstein et al., "Care Taker Role Fatigue," *Nursing Outlook* 29, no. 1 (1981):25-27.

23. Murphy, p. 272.

24. Buckingham, "Public Health Policy," p. 19; Robert Buckingham, "Care of the Dying," *Kansas Journal of Health Concerns* 14, no. 2 (1978): 24; Kennedy, p. 7.

25. Kennedy, p. 8.

26. M. A. Rose, "Problems Families Face in Home Care," *American Journal of Nursing* 76, no. 3 (1976):418; Buckingham, "Hospice," p. 166.

27. Martinson, "Home Care for Children," p. 112; Buckingham, *A Special Kind of Love,* p. 72.

28. Buckingham, *A Special Kind of Love,* p. 71; Martinson, "Home Care for Children," pp. 110 and 112.

## Chapter 5 / The Economics of Home Health Care

1. John Hammond, "Home Health Care Cost Effectiveness: An Overview of the Literature," *Public Health Reports* 94, no. 4 (1979);305-11.

2. Charles Weller, "Home Health Care," *New York State Journal of Medicine* 78, no. 12 (1978):1957-62.

3. Judith La Vor and Marie Callender, "Home Health Cost Effectiveness: What Are We Measuring?" *Medical Care* 14, no. 10 (1976):866-72.

4. G. Harlow Flory, "Medicare Changes Ease Home Health Care Financing," *Pennsylvania Medicine* 84, no. 9 (1981):16-17.

5. Lowell W. Gerson and Owen P. Hughes, "A Comparative Study of the Economics of Home Care," *International Journal of Health Services* 6, no. 4 (1976):543-56.

6. Ibid.

7. Bernard S. Bloom and Priscilla D. Kissick, "Home and Hospital Cost of Terminal Illness," *Medical Care* 18, no. 5 (1980):560-64.

8. Ibid.

9. Flory, pp. 16-17.

10. Philip Buckner et al., "Home Maintenance of the Home Bound Aged: A Pilot Program in New York City," *The Gerontologist* 16, no. 1 (1976): 25-30.

11. Ibid.

12. Ibid.

13. Ibid.

14. C. Carl Pegels, "Institutional versus Noninstitutional Care for the Elderly," *Journal of Health Politics, Policy and Law,* 5, no. 2 (1980):205-12.

15. Ibid.

16. Ibid.

17. Ibid.

18. Ibid.

19. John N. Morris and Hirsch S. Ruchlin, "Cost Benefit Analysis of an Emergency Alarm and Response System: A Case Study of a Long-Term Care Program," *Health Service Research* 16, no. 1 (1981):65-79.

20. Janet I. Brabebill et al., "Pharmacy Department Costs and Patient

Charges Associated with a Home Parenteral Nutrition Program," *American Journal of Hospital Pharmacy* 40, no. 2, (1983):260-62.

21. Michael R. Higgins et al., "Cutting the Costs of Dialysis Using Paid Helpers," *Canadian Medical Association Journal* 123, no. 7 (1980):647-48.

22. Larry Van de Creek, "A Home Hospice Profile," *Journal of Family Practice* 14, no. 1 (1982):53-58.

23. William J. Young, "Third Parties and Home Care RTs: The Frustrating Search for a Little Recognition," *Respiratory Therapy* 8, no. 3 (1978): 53-60.

24. Ibid.

25. Ibid.

26. Jerome Koncel, "Home Health Care Can Be Reimbursed," *Hospitals* 16, no. 53 (1979):44-45.

27. L. R. Jordan and A. B. Doll, "Home Health Care," *American Journal of I. V. Therapy and Clinical Nutrition* (February 1983).

28. James D. Synder and Chris Balew, "Home Health Care: Cost Cutter or Another Expense?" *Physician's Management* 21, no. 9 (1981):73-82.

29. Robert C. Davidson, "The Future of Home Health Agencies," *Journal of Community Health* 4, no. 1 (1978):55-66.

**Chapter 6 / The Making of a Home Health Agency**

1. National League for Nursing, *Type, Length and Cost of Care for Home Health Care*, pub. no. 21-1598 (New York, 1975), p. 3.

2. U.S. Department of Health, Education, and Welfare, *Home Health Care under Medicare*, pub. no. (SS A) 80-10042 (Baltimore, Md., 1979), pp. 1-4.

3. National League for Nursing, *Community Health—Strategies for Change*, pub. no. 21-1493 (New York, 1973), pp. 1-4.

4. Ibid., p. 2.

5. National League for Nursing, *Accreditation of Home Health Agencies: Policies and Procedures*, pub. no. 21-1612 (New York, 1976), p. 3.

6. Ibid., pp. 9-10.

7. National League for Nursing, *Accreditation of Home Health Agencies: Criteria and Guide for Preparing Reports*, pub. no. 21-1306 (New York, 1976), pp. 3-18.

8. National League for Nursing, *Accounting Guidelines for Home Health Agencies*, pub. no. 21-1715 (New York, 1978), pp. iii, 1.

9. National League for Nursing, *Expansion of Home Health Services and the Community Health Service System*, pub. no. 21-1699 (New York), p. iii.

10. Ibid., p. iv.
11. Ibid., p. 4.
12. Ibid., p. 4.

## Chapter 7 / How to Facilitate Home Health Care

1. Jane Emmert Stewart, *Home Health Care* (St. Louis: C.V. Mosby Co., 1978), p. 46. Ms. Stewart sees the HHC triad as consisting of the physician, the nurse, and the homemaker-home health aide. I, on the other hand, regard the family as an integral part of the triad.
2. Ibid., p. 53.
3. Ibid., p. 47.
4. Ibid., p. 46.
5. Cornelia Wolf, "The Challenge of Reviving Home Health Care," in *The Issue Is Leadership,* ed. National League for Nursing, Council of Home Health Agencies and Community Health Services (New York: National League for Nursing, 1975), p. 17.
6. Stewart, p. 47.
7. Ibid., pp. 46 and 48.
8. Virginia Boardman, "Preparation of the Primary Care Nurse," in *The Issue Is Leadership,* p. 65; Stewart, pp. 48-49.
9. Boardman, p. 66; Stewart, p. 50.
10. Boardman, p. 66.
11. Ibid.
12. Stewart, pp. 48-49.
13. Betty J. Ruano, "The Clinical Specialist in Nursing,' in *The Issue Is Leadership,* p. 76; Stewart, p. 52.
14. Robert William Buckingham, "Hospice in a Long-Term Care Facility: An Innovative Pattern of Care," *The Journal of Long-Term Care Administration* 1-2 (1974): 11; Isabelle M. Clifford, in *Home Care: Living with Dying,* ed. Elizabeth R. Prichard et al. (New York: Columbia University Press, 1979), p. 223.
15. Ruth B. Freeman, "Some Observations on the Use of Nurse Practitioners in Community Health Nursing," in *The Issue Is Leadership,* pp. 57 and 61.
16. Ibid., pp. 64 and 66.
17. Nancy Robinson, "The Homemaker-Home Health Aide," in *The Issue Is Leadership,* p. 85.
18. Stewart, p. 65.
19. Ibid., pp. 65 and 67.
20. Ibid., p. 96.

21. Ibid., pp. 96, 97, and 99.
22. Ibid.
23. Ibid., p. 99.
24. Ibid.
25. Ibid., p. 111.
26. Ibid., p. 112.
27. Ibid., p. 119.
28. Ibid., pp. 121-22.
29. Ibid., pp. 90-91.
30. Ibid., p. 91.
31. Ibid., p. 92.
32. Ibid., p. 94.

## Chapter 8 / Home Birth: An Old Practice in Rejuvenation

1. Institute of Medicine and National Research Council, *Research Issues in the Assessment of Birth Settings* (Washington, D.C.: National Academy Press, 1982). pp. 2-3.
2. Abraham Flexner, *Medical Education in the United States and Canada: A Report to the Carnegie Foundation for the Advancement of Teaching* (New York: Carnegie Foundation for the Advancement of Teaching, 1910), p. 117; J. W. Williams, "Medical Education and the Midwife Problem in the United States." *Journal of the American Medical Association* 58 (1912):1-7.
3. Institute of Medicine and National Research Council, pp. 2-3.
4. Jane Lewis, *The Politics of Motherhood* (New York: McGill-Queens University Press, 1980).
5. Institute of Medicine and National Research Council. pp. 2-3.
6. Joyce Cameron, Eileen Sharon Chase, and Sallie O'Neal. "Home Births in Salt Lake County, Utah," *American Journal of Public Health* 69, no. 7 (1979):716-17.
7. Claude A. Burnett, James A. Jones, Judith Rooks, et al., "Home Delivery and Neonatal Mortality in North Carolina," *Journal of the American Medical Association* 244, no. 24 (1980):2741-45.
8. I. D. C. Richards and C. J. Roberts, "The 'at Risk' Infant," Lancet 2, no. 518 (1967):711-13.
9. National Center for Health Statistics, "Annual Summary of Births, Deaths, Marriages and Divorces: United States, 1980," *Monthly Vital Statistics Report* 29, no. 13 (1981):1-31; Oregon Center for Health Statistics, *Oregon Vital Statistics County Data, 1981* (Portland, Oreg.: Department of Human Resources, 1982).

10. L. Mehl, G. H. Peterson, M. Whitt, et al., "Outcomes of Elective Home Births: A Series of 1,146 Cases," *Journal of Reproductive Medicine* 19, no. 5 (1977):281-90.

11. L. Mehl and G. H. Peterson, "Home Birth Versus Hospital Birth," Paper presented at the meeting of the American Public Health Association, Miami, Florida, October 20, 1976.

12. E. Bing and G. Barad, *A Birth in the Family* (New York: Bantam Books, 1973); Sheldon Cherry, *Understanding Pregnancy and Childbirth* (New York: Bobbs-Merrill, 1973).

13. Robert Lans, *Birth Book* (Ben Lomond, Calif.: Genesis Press, 1972; Fritz Leboyer, *Birth Without Violence* (New York: Alfred Knopf, 1975); Martin S. Mahla, Francine Pine, and Alfred Bergmen, *The Psychological Birth of the Human Infant* (New York: Basic Books, 1975); Lewis E. Mehl, "Home Delivery Research Today—A Review," *Women and Health* 1, no. 5 (1976): 3–11; D. Stewart and L. Stewart, eds., *Twenty-First Century Obstetrics Now* (Chapel Hill, N.C.: National Association of Parents and Professionals for Safe Alternatives in Childbirth, 1975).

14. S. Arms, *Immaculate Deception* (Boston: Houghton Mifflin Co., 1975), p. 11.

15. *ASUCSB Bulletin* (San Diego: University of California, April 1979).
16. Ibid.
17. G. D. Adamson, "Health Outcome of Home and Hospital Births," Paper presented at the University of California at San Francisco in a series on Continuing Education in the Health Sciences, The Birth Process: Progress and Problems, May 2, 1981.

18. Sheila Kitzinger and John A. Davis, eds., *The Place of Birth* (New York: Oxford University Press, 1978), p. 42.

## Chapter 9 / The Future of Home Birth in the United States

1. Kevin Krajick, "Home vs. Hospital: Where Are Baby, Mother (and Doctor) Safer?" *The New Physician* 31, no. 7 (1982):15.

2. Ronald R. Rindfuss, "The Implications of the Elective Induction of Labor for the Health of Mothers and Children," in *Obstetrical Practices in the United States,* hearing before the United States Senate Subcommittee on Health and Scientific Research of the Committee on Human Resources, U.S. Senate (Washington, D.C.: U.S. Government Printing Office, 1978), p. 59.

3. R. Goodlin, "Physician Bias in Cesarian Section" (letter), *Journal of the American Medical Association* 249, no. 8 (1983): 1005-6; Rindfuss, p. 71.

4. Rindfuss, p. 52.

5. Kieran O'Driscoll and Michael Foley, "Correlation of Decrease in Perinatal Mortality and Increase in Cesarean Section Rates," *Obstetrics and Gynecology* 61, no. 1 (1983):1.

6. Doris Haine, "Maternity Practices Around the World: How Do We Measure Up?" in *Safe Alternatives in Childbirth*, David Stewart and Lee Stewart, eds. (Chapel Hill, N.C.: National Association of Parents and Professionals for Safe Alternatives in Childbirth, 1976), p. 14.

7. Krajick, p. 18; Ann Oakley, *Women Confined: Toward a Sociology of Childbirth* (New York: Schocken Books, 1980), p. 11; Nancy Mills, "The Lay Midwife," in *Safe Alternatives in Childbirth*, p. 128.

8. Krajick, p. 18; "Birthday at Home: Is It Safe?" *Medical World News* 17, no.8 (1976):105; Claude Burnett, James Jones, Judith Rook, et al., "Home Delivery and Neonatal Mortality in North Carolina," *Journal of the American Medical Association* 244, no. 24 (1980):2743.

9. Stan Bernstein and Ruth Simmons, "Out of Hospital Births in Michigan, 1972–79: Trends and Implications for the Safety of Planned Home Deliveries," *Public Health Reports* 98, no. 2 (1983): 169; "A Time to Be Born" (editorial), *The Lancet* 2, no. 7890 (1974):1183; Rindfuss, p. 166.

10. "No Place Like Home?" (editorial), *The British Medical Journal* (clinical research) 282, no. 6277 (1981):1648; Lee Stewart, "Why Is There a Need for Alternatives in Childbirth?" in *Safe Alternatives in Childbirth*, p. 9.

11. Haine, p. 19.

12. Ibid.; Lewis E. Mehl, "Statistical Outcomes of Home Birth in the United States: Current Status," in *Safe Alternatives in Childbirth*, p. 99.

13. Michael Newton, "What's Best for Newborns and Parents—Giving Birth in the Hospital or at Home?" *Family Health* 9 (1977): 19.

14. Judith Trowell, "Possible Effects of Emergency Cesarean Section on the Mother-Child Relationship," *Early Human Development* 7, no. 1 (1982):49.

## Chapter 10 / Understanding Aging Parents and Grandparents

1. Sophie Reuben and Gloria K. Byrnes, "Helping Elderly Patients in the Transition to a Nursing Home," *Geriatrics* 32, no. 11 (1977):107.

2. Ibid., p. 407.

3. Edith M. Stern and Mabel Ross, *You and Your Aging Parents* (New York: A. A. Wyn, 1952), p. 17.

4. Robert N. Butler, *Why Survive? Being Old in America* (New York: Harper and Row, 1975), p. 419.

5. Arlie Russell Hochschild, *The Unexpected Community* (New Jersey: Prentice-Hall, 1973), p. 91.

6. Ibid.
7. Butler, p. 298.
8. Bertha G. Simos, "Adult Children and Their Aging Parents," *Social Work* 18, no. 3 (1973):81.
9. *Dialogues of Plato,* translated B. Jowett (New York: Clarendon Press, 1953), p. 165.


## Chapter 11 / Home Care for the Elderly

1. Blue Cross Association, "Pilot Program Extends Plans Home Care Coverage," *Blue Cross Consumer Exchange* (February 1978).
2. Helen Kistin and Robert Morris, "Alternatives to Institutional Care for the Elderly and Disabled," *The Gerontologist* 12, no. 2 (1972):141.
3. Neville J. G. Doherty and Barbara C. Hicks, "The Use of Cost-Effectiveness Analysis in Geriatric Day Care," *The Gerontologist* 15, no. 5 (1975):412–13.
4. Ibid.
5. Jean N. Kiernat, "Geriatric Day Hospitals: A Golden Opportunity for Therapists," *American Journal of Occupational Therapy* 30, no. 5 (1976):285.
6. Ibid., p. 286.
7. Connecticut Health Department, *Alternatives to Institutionalization: A Special Report* (Bridgeport: Connecticut Health Department, December 1976), p. 8.


## Chapter 12 / A New Look at Home Care for the Aged

1. Philip W. Brickner, *Home Health Care for the Aged* (New York: Appleton-Century-Cofts, 1978).
2. Theodore H. Koff, *Long Term Care: An Approach to Serving the Frail Elderly* (Boston: Little, Brown and Co., 1982).
3. United States Department of Health, Education, and Welfare, *An Overview of Nursing Home Characteristics* (Washington, D.C.: U.S. Government Printing Office).
4. Robert Butler, "No Place to Live," in *Why Survive? Being Old in America* (New York: Harper and Row, 1975); R. B. Andrew, "Housing for the Elderly: Aspects of Its Central Problem," *The Gerontologist* 3 (1962):110.
5. Donald M. Watkin, "Nutritional Needs of Elderly Intertwined with Other Factors and Attitudes Affecting Health," *Geriatrics* 29, no. 3 (1974):40.
6. Floyd K. Garetz, "Breaking the Dangerous Cycle of Depression and Faulty Nutrition," *Geriatrics* 31, no. 6 (1976):73.

7. W. Latchford, "Nutritional Problems of the Elderly," *Community Health* 16 (1981):145.

8. W. McAllister, "Implementing a Portable Meals Program," *Journal of the American Dietetic Association* 66, no. 4 (1975):375.

9. W. E. Berg, L. Atlas, and J. Zeiger, "Integrated Homemaking Services for the Aged in Urban Neighborhoods,' *The Gerontologist* 14, no. 1 (1974):388.

10. Health Occupations Education, *Home Health Assisting Program Development Guide No. 4* (Albany: University of the State of New York, State Education Department, 1975).

11. Janet Sainer, "Human Services Constraints at State and Local Levels," *The Gerontologist* 23, no. 4 (1983).

12. William W. Lammers, *Public Policy and the Aging* (Washington, D.C.: Congressional Quarterly, 1983), p. 5.

13. Koff, p. 60.

14. Brickner, p. 23; P. E. Ruber, "Home Health Care": It Shows Promise, But...," *Geriatrics* 8, no. 4 (1983):139, 142, and 144.

## Chapter 13 / Group Homes for the Aged

1. L. Trichard, A. Zabow, and L. S. Gillis, "Elderly Persons in Old-Age Homes," *South African Medical Journal* 61, no. 24 (1982):624.

2. L. S. Gillis, R. Elk, L. Trichard, et al., "The Admission of the Elderly to Places of Care: A Socio-Psychiatric Community Survey," *Psychological Medicine* 12, no. 1 (1982):160.

3. Ibid., p. 164.

4. Ibid., p. 160.

5. George Masteron, "Primary Health Care in Residential Homes for the Elderly," *British Medical Journal* 283, no. 6305 (1981):1545.

6. K. Morgan, "Primary Health Care in Residential Homes for the Elderly," *British Medical Journal* 284, no. 6316 (1982):664.

7. Ibid.

8. Trichard, p. 624.

9. Ibid., p. 625.

10. Gillis, p. 625.

11. Trichard, pp. 625-26.

12. M. G. Clarke, A. J. Williams, and P. A. Jones, "A Psychogeriatric Survey of Old People's Homes," *British Medical Journal* 283, no. 6277 (1981): 1307.

13. Sara Simpson, Robert Woods, and Peter Britton, "Depression and Engagement in a Residential Home for the Elderly," *Behavior Research and Therapy* 19 (1981):436.

14. Ibid., p. 437.
15. Ibid., p. 438.
16. Trichard, p. 626.
17. Gillis, p. 163.
18. Ibid., p. 164.
19. Ibid.
20. Ibid.

## Chapter 14 / Home Care for Dying Children

1. Ida M. Martinson, *Home Care for the Dying Child* (New York: Appleton-Century-Crofts, 1976), p. 13.
2. Ida M. Martinson et al., "Facilitating Home Care for Children Dying of Cancer," *Cancer Nursing* 1, no. 1 (1978):41.
3. Anne Heindon, Robert Michielutte, and Richard B. Patterson, "Evaluation of a Home Visitation Program for Families of Children with Cancer," *The American Journal of Pediatrics Hematology/Oncology* 3, no. 3 (1981): 240.
4. Martinson, p. 6.
5. Ibid., p. 13.
6. D. Gay Moldow, Gordon Armstrong, William Henry, and Ida Martinson, "The Cost of Home Care for Dying Children," *Medical Care* 20, no. 11 (1982):1154.
7. Martinson et al., p. 4.
8. Ibid.
9. Ibid.
10. Ibid.

## Chapter 15 / Independent Living for the Physically Disabled

1. C. Beloach and B. Greer, *Adjustment to Severe Disability—A Metamorphosis* (New York: McGraw-Hill, 1981), p. 134.
2. Ibid., p. 142.
3. United States Commission on Civil Rights, *Accommodating the Spectrum of Individual Abilities* (Washington, D.C.: Clearinghouse Publication 81, September 1983), p. 31.
4. Gerber DeJong and Tes Wenber, "Attendant Care as a Prototype Independent Living Services," *Archives of Physical Medicine and Rehabilitation* 60 (October 1979):479.
5. Janet Hart, Mark Moilanen, and Alan S. Bensman, "Transitional Rehabilitation: Another Step toward Community Living," *Rehabilitation Literature* 44, nos. 5-6 (1983):152.

### Chapter 16 / The Marketing of Home Care

1. Andrew J. Riddell, *A Home Health Agency's Approach to Marketing* (New York: National League for Nursing, 1978), pp. 1–2.
2. Evelyn M. Baulch, *Home Care: A Practical Alternative to Extended Hospitalization* (Millbrae, Calif.: Celestial Arts, 1980), p. 10; Hans C. Palmer, "Home Care," in *Long-Term Care: Perspectives from Research and Demonstration*, ed. Ronald J. Vogel and Hans C. Palmer (Washington, D.C.: U.S. Government Printing Office, 1983), p. 341; Drew M. Peterson, "Home Health Care: Whose Decision?" *Assembly of Home Health Agencies; Home Health Agency Concerns Regarding Medicare* (New York: National League for Nursing, 1980), p. 24; Jane Henry Stolten, *Home Care: A Guide to Family Nursing* (Boston: Little, Brown and Co., 1975), p. 1; Louis Barclay Murphy, *The Home Hospital: How a Family Can Cope with Catastrophic Illness* (New York: Basic Books, 1982), p. 4.
3. David Littauer, *Home Care* (Chicago: American Hospital Association, 1961), pp. 9, 100, and 101.
4. Riddell, pp. 2 and 4.
5. Elsie I. Griffith, "Home Health Agencies Today," in *Assembly of Home Health Agencies; Home Health Agency Concerns Regarding Medicare*, p. 6.
6. Theodore Irwin, *Home Health Care: When a Patient Leaves the Hospital* (New York: Public Affairs Committee, no. 560, 1978), p. 4; Palmer, p. 345.
7. Riddell, p. 2.
8. Peterson, p. 135; Irwin, p. 27; U.S. Department of Health, Education, and Welfare, Intradepartmental H.H.C. Policy Working Group, *Home Health Care: A Discussion Paper* (Washington, D.C.: U.S. Government Printing Office, 1979), pp. 9–10.
9. Riddell, p. 6.
10. Irwin. pp. 2, 8, and 10; Littauer, p. 8.
11. Ibid., pp. 13–14.
12. Baulch, p. 159.
13. Ibid., p. 172.
14. Riddell, pp. 3–4; J. A. Sheehan, "Home Care Market: Selling a Concept," *Medical Products Sales* (March 1982):22.
15. Leslie Champlin, "Home Care Market: One Stop Shopping," *Medical Products Sales,* (August 1981):22; Peterson, p. 23.
16. Irwin, p. 27; Riddell, p. 5.
17. Ibid., pp. 5–6; Irwin, p. 5.
18. Sheehan, p. 27.
19. Ibid., pp. 4–6.

20. U.S. Department of Health, Education, and Welfare, Intradepartmental H.H.C. Policy Working Group, pp. 9–12.

21. Ibid., p. 12; Murphy, pp. 3, 14, 15, and 16.

22. Irwin, p. 2; Griffith, pp. 120–21; Littauer, pp. 98 and 100.

23. Irwin, pp. 22 and 24.

24. Griffith, pp. 92 and 97; Irwin, pp. 10, 21, and 22.

25. Ibid., 23.

26. Peterson, p. 133.

27. Ibid., pp. 92 and 130; Riddell, p. 7.

28. Stolten, pp. 1 and 3.

29. Baulch, p. 13.

30. Murphy, p. 5.

## Chapter 17 / Conclusion

1. Ivan Illich, *Deschooling Society* (New York: Harper and Row, 1977), p. 5.

2. Rick J. Carlson, *The End of Medicine* (New York: John Wiley and Sons, 1982), p. 130.

3. Patricia A. Kennedy, *Dying at Home with Cancer* (Springfield, Ill.: Charles Thomas, 1982), p. 6.

4. Ibid.

5. Margaret Cahoon, ed., *Cancer Nursing* (London: Churchill Livingstone, 1982), p. 37; Carlson, pp. 178–79.

6. Nancy Burns, *Nursing and Cancer* (Philadelphia: W.B. Saunders Co., 1982), p. 312; Alan Peter Sager, *Planning Home Care with the Elderly* (Cambridge, Mass.: Ballinger Publishing Co., 1983) p. 41.

7. Anne Minley, *Hospice Alternative* (New York: Basic Books, 1983), p. 121.

8. Burns, p. 3.

9. Carlson, p. 56; Sandra Anderson and Eleanor Bauwers, *Chronic Health Problems* (St. Louis: C.V. Mosby Co., 1981), p. 64.

10. Paul Ramsey, *Ethics at the Edge of Life* (New Haven: Yale University Press, 1978), p. 158.

11. Lisa Mauino, in *Cancer Nursing,* p. 69.

12. Norman Cousins, *Anatomy of an Illness* (New York: W.W. Norton and Co., 1979), p. 29.

13. Kennedy, p. 97.

14. Minley, p. 79.

15. Burns, p. 356.

16. Ibid., p. 358.

17. Ibid., p. 358.

18. John J. Spinetta and Patricia M. Deasy-Spinetta, *Living with Childhood Cancer* (St. Louis: C.V. Mosby Co., 1981), p. 75.

19. Robert Murphy and Leo Reeder, *Psychological Aspects of Cancer* (New York: Raven Press, 1982), p. 26.

20. Stephen Levine and Ondrea Levine, "Learning from Dying," *Medical Self-Care*, 22 (Fall, 1983):14.

21. Carolyn J. Kellog and Barbara P. Sullivan, eds., *Current Perspectives in Oncological Nursing* (St. Louis: C.V. Mosby Co., 1978), p. 8.

22. Ibid.

23. Levine and Levine, p. 12.

24. Burns, p. 102.

25. Levine and Levine, p. 15.

26. Ibid., p. 16.

27. Carlson, pp. 17 and 177.

# SELECT BIBLIOGRAPHY

Anderson, Sandra, and Bauwers, Eleanor. *Chronic Health Problems.* St. Louis: C.V. Mosby Co., 1981.

Arms, S. *Immaculate Deception.* Boston: Houghton Mifflin Co., 1975.

Barnes, MaryLou, and Crutchfield, Carolyn A. *The Patient at Home.* Thorofare, N.J.: Slack Inc., 1973.

Batley, Judith. *The National Health Care Controversy.* New York: Franklin Watts, 1981.

Baulch, Evelyn M. *Home Care: A Practical Alternative to Extended Hospitalization.* Millbrae, Calif.: Celestial Arts, 1980.

BeLoach, C., and Green, B. *Adjustment to Severe Disability—A Metamorphosis.* New York: McGraw Hill, 1981.

Bing, E., and Barad, G. *A Birth in the Family.* New York: Bantam Publications, 1973.

Buckingham, Robert, *A Special Kind of Love: Care of the Dying Child.* New York: Continuum, 1983.

Butler, Robert W., *Why Survive? Being Old in America.* New York: Harper and Row, 1975.

Callahan, James, J., Jr., and Wallack, Stanley S., eds., *Reforming the Long Term Care System.* Lexington, Mass.: D.C. Heath and Co., 1981.

Carlson, Rick J., *The End of Medicine.* New York: John Wiley and Sons, 1982.

Cherry, Sheldon, *Understanding Pregnancy and Childbirth.* New York: Bobbs-Merrill, 1973.

Cousins, Norman, *Anatomy of an Illness.* New York: W.W. Norton and Co., 1979.

Fromstein, Robert H., and Churchill, Jacqueline Curtis. *Psychological Intervention for Hospital Discharge Planning.* Springfield, Ill.: Charles C. Thomas, 1982.

Hochschild, Arlie Russell, *The Unexpected Community.* New Jersey: Prentice-Hall, Inc., 1973.

Illich, Ivan, *Deschooling Society*. New York: Harper and Row, 1977.

Irwin, Theodore, *Home Health Care—When a Patient Leaves the Hospital*. New York: Public Affairs Committee, 1978.

Jenson, F.; Weisbotten, J. G.; and Thomas, M. A. *Medical Care of the Discharged Hospital Patient*. New York: The Commonwealth Fund, 1944.

Johnstone, Margaret. *Home Care for the Strobe Patient: Living in a Pattern*. New York: Churchill Livingstone, 1980.

Kennedy, Patricia A. *Dying at Home with Cancer*. Springfield, Ill.: Charles C. Thomas, 1982.

Kitzner, Sheila, and Davis, John A., eds., *The Place of Birth*. New York: Oxford University Press, 1978.

Kübler-Ross, Elisabeth. *On Death and Dying*. New York: Macmillan Publishing Co., 1969.

Lang, Robert. *Birth Book*. Ben Lomond, Calif.: Genesis Press, 1972.

Leboyer, Fritz. *Birth Without Violence*. New York: Alfred Knopf, 1975.

Lewis, Jane. *The Politics of Motherhood*. New York: McGill-Queens University Press, 1980.

Lipp, M. R. *Respectful Treatment: The Human Side of Medical Care*. New York: Harper and Row, 1977.

Mahler, Martin S.; Pine, Francine; and Bergmen, Alfred. *The Psychological Birth of the Human Infant*. New York: Basic Books, 1975.

Martinson, Ida M. *Home Care for the Dying Child*. New York: Appleton-Century-Crofts, 1976.

_____ et al. "Facilitating Home Care for Children Dying of Cancer." *Cancer Nursing* 1, no. 1 (1978).

_____ et al. "When the Patient Is Dying: Home Care for the Child." *American Journal of Nursing* 77, no. 11 (1977).

Minley, Anne. *The Hospice Alternative*. New York: Basic Books, 1983.

Murphy, Louis Barclay. *The Home Hospital: How a Family Can Cope with Catastrophic Illness*. New York: Basic Books, 1982.

National League for Nursing. *The Issue Is Leadership*. New York: National League for Nursing, 1975.

Papsidero, Joseph A.; Katz, Sidney, Sr.; Kroger, Mary Honora; and Akpom, C. Amechi; eds. *Chance for Change: Implications of a Chronic Disease Module Study*. Lansing: Michigan State University Press, 1979.

Prichard, Elizabeth R.; Collard, Jean; Starr, Janet; Lockwood, Josephine A.; Kutscher, Austin H.; and Seeland, Irene B.; eds., *Home Care: Living with Dying*. New York: Columbia University Press, 1979.

Rose, M. A. "Problems Familes Face in Home Care." *American Journal of Nursing* 76, no. 3 (1976).

Ryder, C. R. *Changing Patterns in Home Care*. (Arlington, Va.: Department of Health, Education, and Welfare, 1967).

Schmidt, Alice M. *The Homemaker's Guide to Home Nursing.* Provo, Utah: Brigham Young University Press, 1976.

Speigal, Alan, and Backhart, Bernard. *Curing and Caring.* New York: Spectrum, 1980.

Stein, Jane J. *Making Medical Choices: Ethics and Medicine in a Technological Age.* Boston: Houghton Mifflin Co., 1978.

Stein, Edith M., and Ross, Mabel. *You and Your Aging Parents.* New York: A.A. Wyn, Inc., 1952.

Stewart, David, and Stewart, Lee, eds., *Safe Alternatives in Childbirth.* Chapel Hill, N.C.: National Association of Parents and Professionals for Safe Alternatives in Childbirth, 1976.

Stewart, Jane Emmert. *Home Health Care.* St. Louis: C.V. Mosby Co., 1978.

Stolten, Jane Henry. *Home Care: A Guide to Family Nursing.* Boston: Little, Brown and Co., 1975.

Tinkham, Catherine, and Voorhies, Eleanor F. *Community Health Nursing: Evolution and Process.* New York: Appleton-Century-Crofts, 1977.

United States Commission on Civil Rights. *Accommodating the Spectrum of Individual Abilities.* Washington: Clearinghouse Publication 81, September, 1983.

Wensley, Edith. *Nursing Service Without Walls: A Call to Action to All Communities Coast to Coast.* New York: National League for Nursing, 1963.